CHIROPRACTIC
FIRST

The Fastest Growing Healthcare Choice. . . Before Drugs or Surgery

Terry A. Rondberg, D. C.

The
CHIROPRACTIC
Journal

CHIROPRACTIC FIRST
The Fastest Growing Healthcare Choice...
Before Drugs Or Surgery

Published by:
The Chiropractic Journal

Library of Congress Catalog Number: 95-92445
ISBN: 0-9647168-2-8

44 45 46 47 48 49 50 51 52 53 54 55 56

Photographs of Daniel D. Palmer and Bartlett J. Palmer with permission from the Palmer College of Chiropractic.

I dedicate this book
To my mother, Lois Lee Rondberg, for introducing me to
chiropractic,
To my father, Daniel Rondberg, for always supporting me
in my ideals,
To Cindy, my wife and my best friend and
To my daughters, Brooke and Shannon,
Thank you for all your love and understanding.

WHAT THE READERS ARE SAYING

"Humanity desperately needs a solution to the health care crisis — Chiropractic First provides that answer in a clear and uncompromising way. Every D.C. should make this book a 'must read' for new patients."

—Christopher Kent, D.C.
President of the Council on Chiropractic Practice (CCP)

"Extremely educational and thoroughly enjoyable... Dr. Rondberg writes in a clear, concise style that is easy to follow and hold the reader's attention. He takes the reader through a step-by-step account of how the body works, what chiropractic is, and how chiropractic can enhance our health and wellness."

—Pamela Hertzberg
Chiropractic Assistant (CA)

"...bringing a new, clearer dynamic insight to Chiropractors, patients and the public, your book is on my must-read list. Everyone better read this book now!"

—Guy Riekeman, D.C.
President, Palmer Chiropractic University

"...an excellent book to start patients on the road to help begin their transformation."

—Greg Stanley
CEO, Whitehall Management

"Clear, concise and inspirational... every chiropractic patient needs to know this essential information to make better decisions about their health."

—William Esteb
CEO, Patient Media

"The book echoes the classic format of a new patient orientation, providing details of information that all chiropractors wish to disseminate to the general public. Reader friendly both in content and style, the writing technique is well geared to the non-scientific background as an aid in educating both patients and non-patients alike."

—Steven Shochat, D.C.
Director, Cactus Flower Wellness Center

About the Author

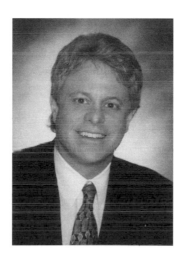

DR. TERRY A. RONDBERG is a prominent leader in the chiropractic profession. He started private practice in 1975 after graduating from Logan College of Chiropractic. Over the next fifteen years he helped thousands of patients in his offices in St. Louis, Missouri and Phoenix, Arizona.

Reaching thousands wasn't enough for Dr. Rondberg. He knew that throughout the country, around the world, there were millions of others who had not yet experienced the power of chiropractic firsthand. Sadly, he also knew that there were millions more who probably never would have that opportunity. They were either cut off from chiropractic care because of unfair insurance practices or they were led to believe that medical treatment was the only avenue to health.

These are the people Dr. Rondberg wanted to reach through an intensive campaign of public education and political action. In 1986, he founded The Chiropractic Journal, a monthly newspaper distributed to every chiropractor and chiropractic student in the world. He uses the pages of his phenomenally successful publication to help build a stronger profession and safeguard it from its enemies.

In the years since he has published The Chiropractic Journal, he has seen the chiropractic profession achieve many of its goals, including a victory in the Wilk vs. AMA law suit, and recognition by numerous government agencies.

In 1989, he widened his horizon even more and founded the World Chiropractic Alliance, a non-profit "watchdog" organization dedicated to promoting a vertebral subluxation-free world. Time and again, the organization has led the fight to protect the consumers' right to choose chiropractic as their first choice in health care. With massive public relations efforts, he has won chiropractic support from people around the world, and has helped inform millions of individuals about the philosophy, art and science of chiropractic.

Reflecting both the depth of his knowledge and the enthusiasm of his convictions, Dr. Rondberg has become a popular speaker at chiropractic conferences, conventions and seminars. A prolific writer, he has also authored numerous publications and articles on chiropractic for both the profession and the public.

TABLE OF CONTENTS

CHIROPRACTIC

By B. J. Palmer

We chiropractors work with the subtle substance of the soul. We release the prisoned impulses, a tiny rivulet of force, that emanates from the mind and flows over the nerves to the cells and stirs them to life. We deal with the magic power that transforms common food into living, loving, thinking clay; that robes the earth with beauty, and hues and scents the flowers with the glory of the air.

In the dim, dark distant long ago, when the sun first bowed to the morning star, this power spoke and there was life, it quickened the slime of the sea and the dust of the earth and drove the cell to union with its fellows in countless living forms. Through eons of time it finned the fish and winged the bird and fanged the beast. Endlessly it worked, evolving its forms until it produced the crowning glory of them all. With tireless energy it blows the bubble of each individual life and then silently, relentlessly dissolves the form and absorbs the spirit into itself again.

And yet you ask "Can chiropractic cure appendicitis or the flu?" Have you more faith in a knife or a spoonful of medicine than in the power that animates the living world?

Chapter 1

"ADJUSTING TO A BETTER LIFE"

I had only been in practice about a year when I first met Mrs. Hoffman. She was recently divorced and working as a waitress to support her children. During our initial consultation, she complained of back pain and said that her back started hurting when she was lifting heavy trays of food. I explained that I adjusted the spine to help the overall body operate at its peak efficiency not directly to alleviate back pain but to correct any nerve interference I found. I told her that often, when I make an adjustment, the patient's back pain disappears. It didn't matter what symptom or condition a person had, he or she would benefit from the correction of nerve interference, resulting in improved nerve supply.

Mrs. Hoffman also asked if I thought I could help her son, Richie, who was "in really bad shape." I said I could usually help "if the patient is alive and has a nerve system." Hope was reflected in her eyes.

Richie was one of seven-year-old twin boys. His brother, Johnny, was just fine, healthy and active. Richie, however, was a different story. He was dying. He'd been seen by seventeen different doctors and not one of them could agree on a diagnosis. In seven years, over thirty-seven different medications had been prescribed for him. He was in the hospital twice for tests and observation. Each time, his stay had been extended and the family's insurance had paid tens of thousands of dollars for Richie's medical expenses. (Now, the family had no insurance because Mr. Hoffman had stopped paying the premiums after the divorce.) The last time he was hospitalized, the baffled doctors felt Richie's condition was hopeless and sent him home with instructions that his mother should make him as comfortable as possible until his death. Currently, Richie was taking five different medications, including the drug Phenobarbital, which is used to control seizures.

Mrs. Hoffman received this dire verdict about a week before she came to see me for her back pain.

After listening to her story, I told her I would examine Richie for nerve interference, and she was not to worry about payment. I referred to the sign in our waiting room which said: "we accept all patients regardless of their condition or financial ability to pay."

When I saw Richie, I must admit I was quite shocked by his physical condition. Mrs. Hoffman had to carry him in her arms into my office. Because of his condition, he had never been able to wear shoes and was dressed only in shorts and a t-shirt. He seemed to have no body or facial hair and his frail body was covered with sores from head to toe. On his legs, the sores were so profuse that I couldn't see any healthy skin. Furthermore, he was so drugged from the five different medications he was taking that his eyes were rolling back in his head. Richie really looked closer to death than anyone I had ever seen. His brother Johnny had come with them and the contrast between the two children made Richie's situation all the more dramatic.

It was difficult to examine the boy. I was so moved by his condition, I actually had to leave the examining room to regain my composure. When I returned and examined him, I explained to his mother that Richie had nerve interference in his neck. I told her I would adjust him every day for awhile. Even though it was illegal for me to give advice about medications, I went so far as to tell her that if Richie were my child, I would slowly try to reduce his medications.

We agreed that I would adjust Mrs. Hoffman and both her sons for five dollars a week. I had found nerve interference in Johnny's spine even though he said he felt great. I wanted to adjust him before he developed symptoms.

After I'd been working with the family for about six weeks, I began to get discouraged. I didn't see any real change in Richie's condition and I wondered if his mother noticed this too, and felt disappointed.

When I questioned her as to whether or not she thought the adjustments were helping, I have never forgotten what she said to me. I was a young doctor then, but many years later, I still carry her message of faith with me. Mrs. Hoffman said:

"When I first came to you, I also suffered with severe headaches and menstrual cramps I never told you about. I was taking a lot of medication which I now no longer need. I feel great except for my back, but it seems improved.

"You explained how the power that made my body is the only power that could heal it and I knew you were talking about God.

5

I understand that it may be too late for Richie because he's been sick so long, but, if you give up on him, I have no other place to go for help.

"Your adjustments have already helped me so much, I just know that if it's God's will for Richie to recover, then he is going to get better. Please don't give up, Dr. Rondberg. "

How could I do anything but agree to continue the adjustments? I cast aside my own discouragement and lack of faith and made a promise to myself that I would never again doubt the ability of my adjustments or the hope they offered.

The very next week, the miracle began to unfold. Richie's mother excitedly showed me some areas of clear skin where earlier there had only been open bloody sores. (She had gradually reduced his medication.) The child continued to make progress and, at the end of eight weeks of care, it was obvious that his body was healing at an amazing rate. He was excited about the hair fuzz growing on top of his head. Furthermore, he was walking into my office now, and he was proudly wearing his first pair of shoes.

It took several more months for Richie to be completely healed. Finally, the only reminders of his condition were areas of skin that were marked with a pinkish coloration where the open sores had been.

I never found out the correct name for Richie's medical condition because none of the experts could agree on a diagnosis. The only thing Mrs. Hoffman and I cared about was that Richie got his life back. It was stunning proof that with an improved spinal structure, the potential for a healthy body and normal function can return.

And I will always be grateful for the lesson I learned

about not giving up on any patient regardless of his or her disease. I have always limited my practice objective to specific adjusting for the correction of nerve interference. I gave each of my patients the opportunity to receive care that would help eliminate the interference to their body's natural expression of Innate Wisdom.

❄ ❄ ❄

OPTIMAL HEALTH CARE

If you could create the most satisfying healing system imaginable, what would you recommend? Most of us would want a natural method, one that utilizes the body's own abilities to promote internal healing and on-going wellness. Dangerous drugs would not be used and frightening surgeries would not be performed.

If it sounds like such a system is too good to be true, you are in for a pleasant surprise. There is such a system of healing. While the roots of manipulation are in antiquity, true chiropractic began in 1895. To date, millions of people have benefited from this non-medical, drug-free health care.

Chiropractic is the largest natural primary health care profession in the world. It's one of the most praised yet most misunderstood of all the health care disciplines, despite the fact that more than twenty-five million Americans utilize it each year. It's practiced by 50,000 doctors around the world and is licensed in every state in the Union. In accredited colleges in America, Japan, England, Australia, Canada, France and South Africa more than 7500 students are studying this discipline.

❄ ❄ ❄

HISTORY OF CHIROPRACTIC

If you think that chiropractic is a new science, it is. However, you will be surprised to know the first pictures depicting spinal manipulation were discovered in prehistoric cave paintings in Point le Merd in southwestern France. They may have been crude, non-specific attempts to manipulate the spine, but these early historical records date back to 17,500 B.C. The ancient Chinese were using manipulation in 2700 B.C, Greek papyruses from 1500 B.C. gave directions for solving low-back problems by maneuvering the legs. We also know that the ancient Japanese, Egyptians, Babylonians, Hindus, Tibetans and Syrians all practiced spinal manipulation. Even in Tahiti, there is evidence that manipulative therapy has been used for centuries.

Historical records in Egypt reveal that men and women were stronger and healthier when their backs were straight instead of twisted. The Egyptians were very concerned with correcting the spine.

Ancient American Indian hieroglyphics showed *back walking* (that is, walking on the back of a patient) being practiced as a method of curing the sick. The Sioux, Winnebago and Creek Indians in North America all left records of manipulation and healing. In Mexico and Central America, the Mayan, Aztec, Toltec, Tarascan, and Zoltec Indians routinely used manipulation. The South American Incas were sophisticated enough to develop manipulation into a well-defined and well-documented art.

Hippocrates was a Greek physician who died in 377 B.C. He wrote over seventy books on healing and was a proponent of spinal manipulation. He believed that only

8

nature could heal and it was the physician's duty to remove any obstruction that would prevent the body from healing.

"Get knowledge of the spine, for this is the requisite for many diseases."

Hippocrates, 460-377 BC.

Hippocrates believed that the essence of life and the natural healing ability of the body were the result of a *vital spirit*. That same concept of "vitalism" occurred throughout ancient writings. In the Twentieth Century, vitalism was replaced by the idea of an Innate Intelligence.

Herodotus, a contemporary of Hippocrates, gained fame curing diseases by correcting spinal abnormalities through therapeutic exercises. If the patient was too weak to exercise, Herodotus would manipulate the patient's spine. The philosopher Aristotle was critical of Herodotus' tonic-free approach because, "he made old men young and thus prolonged their lives too greatly." This would be considered a benefit today but it was disconcerting in early Greece where the life expectancy was very limited—not more than three decades.

In Greece crude mechanical devices were invented to stretch the spine and correct dislocations. Archaeologists have also uncovered pictures of Greek patients being hung upside down by their heels. Physicians also walked on patient's backs to correct spinal deviations.

In Rome, by the Second Century A.D., Claudius Galen taught the proper positions and relations of the vertebrae and the spinal column. Galen was known as the *Prince of Physicians*, a title he was given after he aligned the neck

9

vertebrae of a well-known Roman scholar whose right hand was paralyzed. Once the vertebra was aligned, nerve transmission was restored and the scholar was able to use his hand again. Galen's reputation was made!

The skills of spinal manipulation were handed down within families and almost every village boasted a "bonesetter" who could cure by straightening the spine. In both Eastern and Western cultures, manipulation of soft tissues or massage were recognized as a useful component in health care.

Crude types of manipulation continued all over the world until Daniel David (D.D.) Palmer discovered the correct specific spinal adjustment. It was his son, B. J. Palmer, who later developed it into the modern philosophy, art and science of chiropractic we are familiar with today. D.D. Palmer thought that commonly used drugs and potions were actually toxic and created stress for ill patients. He was more interested in finding the cause of the disease and eliminating it through natural means.

"I am not the first person to replace subluxated vertebrae, but I do claim to be the first person to replace displaced vertebrae by using the spinous and transverse processes as levers...and to develop the philosophy and science of chiropractic adjustments."

D.D. Palmer, Discoverer of Chiropractic

D.D. Palmer was born in Ontario, Canada, in 1845, He moved to the United States when he was twenty-years-old. He spent the years after the Civil War teaching school, raising bees and selling sweet raspberries in the Iowa and Illinois river towns along the bluffs on either side of the Mississippi River.

While living in What Cheer, Iowa in 1885, D.D. became familiar with the work of Paul Caster, a magnetic healer who had some success in Ottumwa. D.D. moved his family to Burlington, near Ottumwa, and learned the techniques of magnetic healing. This was a common therapy. At the time practitioners used the body's natural magnetic properties for healing purposes. Two years later he moved his family again, this time to Davenport, Iowa, where he opened the Palmer Cure & Infirmary.

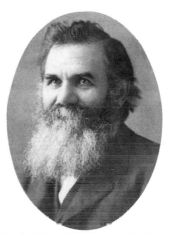

Daniel David Palmer. (D D)

On September 18, 1895, D.D. Palmer performed his first adjustment on a janitor, Harvey Lillard, who had been deaf for seventeen years. The man's hearing returned, and because of the success of Palmer's spinal adjustment, the modern recorded history of chiropractic began.

Here is the description of this event in D.D. Palmer's own words.

"Harvey Lillard...could not hear the racket of a wagon on the street or the ticking of a watch. I made inquiry as to the cause of his deafness and was informed that when he was exerting himself in a cramped, stooping position, he felt something give way in his back and immediately became deaf.

"An examination showed a vertebra racked from its normal position. I reasoned that if that vertebra was replaced, the man's hearing should be restored. With this object in view, a half hour's talk persuaded Mr. Lillard to allow me to replace it. I racked it

11

into position by using the spinous process as a lever, and soon the man could hear as before.

"There was nothing accidental about this as it was accomplished with an object in view, and the result expected was obtained. There was nothing 'crude' about this adjustment; it was specific, so much so that no other Chiropractor has equaled it."

Over the succeeding months, other patients came to him with diverse problems including flu, sciatica, migraine headaches, stomach complaints, epilepsy and heart problems. D.D. Palmer found each of these conditions responded well to the adjustments which he was calling "hand treatments." Later he coined the term *chiropractic*, from the Greek words, *Chiro*, meaning (hand) and *practic*, meaning (practice or operation). He renamed his clinic the Palmer School & Infirmary of Chiropractic.

The term "Infirmary" (implying medicinal treatment) was confusing because none of the patients were given medicines of any kind. They hadn't undergone surgery. Under Palmer's care fevers broke, pain ended, infections healed, vision improved, stomach disorders disappeared, and of course, hearing returned. Palmer knew what to do for these people. What he didn't know was *why* his treatments were so effective.

Often surprised at the effectiveness of his adjustments, D.D. Palmer returned to his studies of anatomy and physiology to learn more about the vital connection between the spine and one's health. He realized spinal adjustments were correcting vertebral subluxations, (nerve interference), that was causing the patients' complaints. Based on the body's Innate ability to heal itself—and aided by the practitioner's ability to correct the nerve interference—chiropractic often brings an end to needless suffering from pain and discomfort in natural ways unknown in any other health discipline. It is one of the most powerful and effective healing methods available today.

At first, even though it proved to be a successful way of healing the body, chiropractic adjustments were not readily accepted.

Years after Harvey Lillard's hearing was restored, the news media delighted in vilifying the pioneer chiropractor. D.D. Palmer was labeled a "charlatan" and a "crank on magnetism." The medical community, afraid of his success and discouraged by its own failure to heal diseases, joined the crusade and wrote letters to the editors of local papers, openly criticizing his methods and accusing him of practicing medicine without a license.

D.D. Palmer defended himself against the doctors' attacks by presenting arguments against the medical procedures of vaccination and surgery. He also cautioned against introducing medicine into the body saying it was often unnecessary and even harmful.

In 1905, the medical establishment won a minor victory when they conspired to have D.D. Palmer indicted for practicing medicine without a license. He was sentenced to 105 days in jail and was required to pay a $350 fine. At first, he argued with the judge and refused to pay the fine. (The local newspapers gave alot of coverage to this incident.) After serving twenty-three days of his sentence, however, he paid the fine and was released.

From 1906 to 1913, D.D. Palmer published two books, *The Science of Chiropractic* and *The Chiropractor's Adjuster.* He died in Los Angeles at the age of sixty-eight, after being stricken by typhoid fever. The world owes much to D.D. Palmer. His son B.J. once stated that he felt his father D.D. had done more for mankind than any other single individual and should be compared with other great men such as Thomas Edison.

"I desired to know why one person was ailing and his associate, eating at the same table, working in the same shop...was not. Why? What difference was there in the two persons that caused one to have [disease] while his partner...escaped? Why?

D.D. Palmer, Discoverer of Chiropractic

B. J. PALMER

It was D.D. Palmer's son, Bartlett Joshua Palmer, who is credited with *developing* chiropractic. Born in 1881, B.J., as he was always called, was a prolific author and speaker who was in great demand by audiences worldwide. He had an extraordinary gift as a salesman and his product was chiropractic.

By all accounts, B.J. was as much of a character as his father. He loved to tell stories which were more than a little embellished to make them more entertaining and he thoroughly enjoyed talking to the people who eagerly gathered around him. Even though B.J. had seen very little of his father while he was growing up, when they did get together, they discovered they had similar temperaments and often clashed violently. One time after an argument, D.D. abruptly packed up and moved from Davenport to Portland, Oregon, where he opened the Pacific College of

Chiropractic. The senior Palmer then went on to Santa Barbara, California, to establish another chiropractic clinic, leaving B.J. to cope with the struggling school in Iowa.

Like most great men, B.J. is remembered for his many idiosyncrasics, several of which were embarrassing to his family. He was very adamant about going to bed early in the evening so he could rise at five in the morning to spend several hours writing. Promptly at nine, even if guests were present, he would loosen his tie, take off his shoes, carry them upstairs, and announce that the evening was over—at least as far as he was concerned.

When he went to bed, it was imperative his head was pointed toward the North Pole and his feet to the south. This was how he felt he got the most restful sleep, as he felt the earth's currents would flow through him properly. This belief was so strong that even when he traveled, he would rearrange the hotel furniture to accommodate this need, no matter how late the hour or how inconvenient the restructuring of the room.

Before air-conditioning became commonplace, B.J. would go to bed on the screened-in porch wearing a nightshirt he had soaked in cold water. He believed the evaporation of the water cooled him naturally.

On the third floor of B.J.'s home, he and his father kept their renowned collection of human spines. The spinal columns were hung in rows along the walls and provided an invaluable resource for students at the Palmer School of Chiropractic— as well as endless amusement for B.J.'s son, David, and other youngsters in the neighborhood. As a young boy, David was often asked to perform for company by reciting from memory the 206 bones in the body. This was an accomplishment B.J. felt was more important than

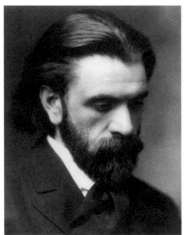

Bartlett Joshua Palmer, (BJ)

playing a musical instrument or memorizing poetry.

B.J. never tasted alcohol, but he did chain-smoke cheap cigars which were manufactured in West Davenport. He only smoked expensive cigars when they were given to him as a gift. While B.J. Palmer was a man of somewhat unorthodox habits, he was the perfect person to carry on his father's work and defend the fledgling profession against its detractors. Because of his efforts, chiropractic survived and was rightfully acknowledged as bringing relief and maintaining health without first resorting to medications.

B. J. felt a deep concern for his father's clinic and infirmary and felt responsible for continuing the school from which he, himself, had graduated in 1902. From the time of his graduation, he became a teacher at the school and also had a private chiropractic practice. In 1905, he moved the school and clinic to a large Victorian home on Brady Street Hill in Davenport, Iowa. The building was partitioned to provide living quarters for B.J. and his young wife, Mabel, who had graduated that same year from the Palmer School. The house also included sleeping quarters for the students and classrooms in the basement.

Through his own efforts, B.J. became a highly educated person who was respected by the civic and financial leaders in Davenport. Under his picture in the gallery of distinguished citizens of Davenport, a plaque reads:

"B. J. Palmer, world renowned as spokesman-developer of his father's discovery of chiropractic. Famed educator, traveler, author, radio-television pioneer (WOC-radio and TV), among the nation's first. President, Palmer College of Chiropractic, 1905-1961."

B.J. Palmer believed that nothing was impossible if you worked hard enough. He used to say: "Only the hen can make money by laying around." He developed the chiropractic philosophy, art and science into a profession at a time when it was little more than a loosely knit structure.

He enabled the Palmer college graduates to be licensed and qualified to practice chiropractic. During the 1920s, the school enrollment was over 2000 students. While other chiropractic schools were springing up all over the world, not one of them was as large as Palmer College.

B.J. Palmer has been described as controversial, visionary, outspoken, eccentric, energetic, single-minded and opinionated. Every one of these terms is appropriate. No one else traveled as much, fought as many court battles, or successfully introduced as much legislation to improve the profession. In 1926, he became president of the International Chiropractors Association. He held the position until his death in 1961. During those years, he fought to have chiropractors licensed by separate licensing boards, all the while carrying on a public feud with Morris Fishbein who was the editor of the *Journal of the American Medical Association*.

In 1910, B.J. advocated the use of Wilhelm Roentgen's invention, the X-ray machine, as a valid tool in the practice of chiropractic. Within the faculty there was a divided philosophy about the use of equipment of any sort. Some of them were so infuriated that they left Palmer College to form their own training facility which they named Universal Chiropractic College. To add fuel to the fire, D.D. Palmer chose to ally himself with the new school, as a slap in the face to his son. D.D. had never forgiven his son for following the advice of his attorney. When D.D. was put in jail four years earlier, the attorney advised that the school's assets be put in his wife's name to protect them. Eventually Universal Chiropractic College closed and was forgotten.

One of B.J.'s strongest weapons in the battle to defend and validate chiropractic was the fledgling medium, commercial radio. By 1922, he and his family had moved away from the school to an imposing residence further up the Brady Street Hill. Inspired by his son David's fascination with ham radio, B.J. bought a 250-watt amateur radio station. He called it WOC (Wonders of Chiropractic) and it became the keystone of the Palmer Communications empire. At first, the station was a family run affair but it soon became the first 500-watt radio station in the United States. In 1927, it became the western most link of the tiny new NBC network. B.J. became so proficient at using the new medium to move people to action, that he wrote a book, *Radio Salesmanship*, which became an essential textbook for anyone in the industry.

After his death, the *Davenport Times* said that B.J.: "...observed that the most effective announcers were those who used as few words as possible to get their point across, and who adopted a positive attitude." Former President Ronald Reagan was employed by B.J. as a radio announcer at WOC.

B.J. loved epigrams and slogans which he collected and shared with others by painting them on walls, stairwells and chimneys all around the campus. He had two sayings that he felt were particularly meaningful: *"The world makes a path for the man who knows where he is going."* And *"Early to bed, early to rise, work like hell and advertise, makes a man healthy, wealthy and wise."* While many of these sayings were his own, B.J. had a special fondness for the words of Mark Twain, Abraham Lincoln, Zane Grey and Teddy Roosevelt.

Earl Ackerman managed the Blackhawk Hotel in Davenport and he was a good friend of B.J. Palmer. He wrote: *"Like his father, B.J. subscribed wholeheartedly to the idea of inner intelligence, the 'Innate,' as they called it. I don't think you could talk to B.J. within a period of 48 hours, say, when he wouldn't mention the word 'Innate' at least a half-dozen times. It was a part of his teaching. He thought that each of us has the 'Innate' within us and that it controls what we do as well as our health. Still, each of us is responsible for what we do, for living a life of accomplishment, but in a way, this all comes from within ourselves."*

Today every Doctor of Chiropractic owes B. J. Palmer a great debt. Without B.J.'s relentless work over his lifetime, the profession of chiropractic would have ended in 1913, along with the passing of D.D. Palmer, instead of flourishing as we enter the 21st century.

THINK! SPEAK! ACT POSITIVE! I AM! I WILL! I CAN! I MUST!

B.J. Palmer, D.C.

MODERN CHIROPRACTIC

THE CHIROPRACTIC PRACTICE OBJECTIVE: The professional practice objective of chiropractic is to correct vertebral subluxations also referred to as nerve interference, in a safe and effective manner. The correction of nerve interference is not considered to be a specific cure for any particular symptom or disease. It is applicable to any patient who exhibits nerve interference regardless of the presence or absence of symptoms or disease.

Today, chiropractic has come a long way from D.D. Palmer's practice in Davenport, Iowa. Specifically, the chiropractor determines the presence of nerve interference and helps the body correct itself by introducing a force in a prescribed manner. Contrary to popular misinformation, the Doctor of Chiropractic (D.C.) doesn't force the misaligned vertebrae back into place but he or she facilitates the body's correction of nerve interference.

During the adjustment, the subluxated vertebrae are unlocked and released from their misaligned positions. The body's inborn intelligence is called upon to shape the spine. When this happens, the vertebrae return to their proper alignment and the normal nerve supply is restored. This allows one to achieve maximum healing potential with a complete nerve supply.

This book, explains what chiropractic is, how it works and what it can do for you and your family. In no way am I suggesting that you should never consult a medical physician. There are surgeries that must be performed, and wounds, broken bones and internal injuries that require medical treatment.

However, you will realize that when confronted with a physical problem, your safest and most effective first choice for general health care should be a chiropractor. You will understand why medicine should be used as the last resort—when the body cannot heal itself without intervention.

Wisdom dictates that you begin the healing process with conservative care that doesn't cause any side effects.

My recommendation:

Chiropractic first, drugs second, and surgery last.

❄ ❄ ❄

DON'T LET YOUR SPINE GET ON YOUR NERVES

The purpose of chiropractic care is the correction of nerve interference. Nerve interference promotes sickness and disease. It robs our vitality and weakens our immune system.

The spinal column consists of twenty-four small bones called vertebrae. Seven of these are located in the neck. Twelve are found in the mid-back and five are in the lower back. The vertebrae stack one on top of the other, and when you look at them from front to back, they form a straight line.

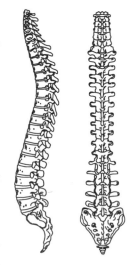

It's very rare to find someone with a spine that's perfectly aligned. In most people, the spine curves slightly

21

to the right or the left and sometimes, one or more of the vertebrae are twisted or rotated.

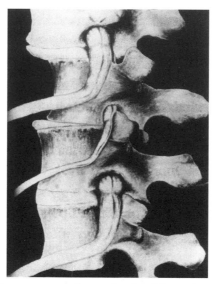

This is one type of vertebral subluxation (spinal nerve interference) — the "silent killer."

When the vertebrae are misaligned, the flow of messages from the brain to all the other cells in the body is distorted. This type of nerve interference creates dis-organization of bodily processes and dis-ease. This misalignment of the vertabrae can often exist undetected and slowly undermine one's health.

DISEASE OR DIS-EASE?

The word *disease*, is a combination of *dis* and *ease*. *Dis* is a prefix meaning "apart from" and *ease* meaning a "state of balance." It follows then that dis-ease is a lack of comfort, a loss of harmony in the system. When there is a lack of harmony in music, the musician adjusts the notes to complement one another and "work well together." That's exactly what an adjustment to correct or reduce nerve interference can do—restore body harmony.

Unlike music, where discord is immediately apparent, damage from nerve interference is not so obvious at first.

The unfortunate aspect of this "dis-ease" is that it need not be painful to silently destroy the body's health and well-being. Gradually, the body's life support systems begin to fail and the ability to live a full life diminishes. Nerve interference is often referred to as a *silent killer*, because it may be present for many years before symptoms arise. It can quietly, painlessly undermine your health before any major warning signs appear.

The causes of nerve interference are numerous and often, unavoidable. They can be caused at birth, if the delivery is difficult or requires the use of forceps. Many births result in subluxations. Children, during the critical growing years, fall while learning to walk. In later years, they engage in activities like skate boarding or surfing and many other kinds of sports which can cause subluxations. Other spinal problems can be caused by a junk food diet or having poor sleeping positions. Many seemingly harmless activities can disturb the integrity of the nerve system.

As adults, many things can weaken the spine, and cause nerve interference. This list includes: sports accidents, automobile collisions, falls in the house, bad posture, emotional stress, dental problems, pushing ourselves past our limits, alcohol and drug abuse or even carrying heavy briefcases or handbags on a daily basis. We've reached a point where nerve interference is epidemic in our population. To ignore it and not have your spine checked regularly by a chiropractor is to invite disease to overwhelm your body and impair the quality of your life. In later chapters, we'll be exploring the connection between your spine and various physical conditions we tend to consider an unavoidable part of our human condition. You'll understand the vital role your spine plays in your life, and gain new insights on how you can promote and maintain good health, with less fear of needing dangerous chemicals and/or invasive surgery.

"To take in a new idea you must destroy the old, let go of old opinions, to observe and conceive new thoughts. To learn is but to change your opinion."

B.J. Palmer, D.C.

A doctor of chiropractic is uniquely trained to locate and help correct nerve system interference which promotes the body's natural healing ability.

Chapter 2

CHIROPRACTIC-101

To understand chiropractic, one must have a basic understanding about how the body functions. This chapter and the next will explain our marvelous machine, the body.

From the time you were born, your Inner Wisdom has known exactly how to keep you healthy and alive. It knows how fast your heart should beat, how often your lungs need to breathe, how to digest food and how to eliminate waste. There are millions of details controlled by your Inner Wisdom to keep this marvelous machine in prime functioning condition.

". . .a kind of super intelligence exists in each of us, infinitely smarter and possessed of technical know-how far beyond our present understanding."

Lewis Thomas, M.D.

Every living organism in our world possesses what chiropractors call Innate Intelligence. The body machine comes out of the "factory" fully able to function, as long it has regular fuel and adequate maintenance.

Innate Intelligence sends instructions to every organ and cell in your body through the nerve system housed by the vertebrae. However, unless your spinal vertebrae are correctly aligned, those instructions can't be received and followed properly. The result is "dis-ease" and dysfunction.

❄ ❄ ❄

THE PHILOSOPHY OF CHIROPRACTIC

While the word *philosophy* may bring to mind ancient Greeks or bearded scholars in dusty libraries, the philosophy of health is a vibrant study that influences how we live. It helps us make critical choices about how we treat our bodies.

Too often, people respond to every symptom by gulping down pills to alleviate the discomfort. When they catch a cold, they buy an over-the-counter remedy from the drugstore. If they gain a few pounds, they head for the diet pills. When they feel tired, they take pills to stay awake and when they want to sleep, there's a pill to take for that, too. There's a bottle of pills to combat headaches and another for irregularity and still another for diarrhea. If you have a symptom, the drug companies have a remedy. The message to the consumer is, whatever is wrong, just pop a pill and you'll be fine. We call this the "Medical Philosophy of Disease. "

Every one of us has symptoms from time to time. When something goes wrong in the body, we get a rash, feel pain or experience discomfort in any one of a hundred ways. The body's warning system is at work. Like the red lights on your car's dashboard, symptoms tell you it's time to check something in your internal machinery. For the followers of the Medical Philosophy of Disease, these warnings are treated by attempting to fix the symptoms and not the cause. These people believe something from the outside will change something on the inside. That state of mind is dangerous to one's health.

Let's go back to the car analogy. Say the oil light comes on. What are you going to do? Pull into your nearest gas station and put a quart of oil in the engine or are you going to disconnect the light so you won't see it? The logical answer doesn't require much thought. Back to your body. If you get a pain in your head, are you going to check out the cause and correct it? Or are you going to take a pain killer and assume the problem is gone because the symptom has been alleviated?

"Each patient carries his own doctor inside him. They come to us not knowing that truth. We are at our best when we give the doctor who resides within each patient a chance to work."

Albert Schweitzer, M.D.

When you realize your body is somewhat similar to a machine, then it's obvious what the answer has to be. You recognize the need to fix the internal mechanism so the machine is working well again. That's the Philosophy of Health. It's the belief that health comes from within. A properly functioning body can do everything naturally that pills attempt to do chemically. Furthermore, the body knows when to heal, how to heal and when to stop healing and go back on maintenance.

If you cut your hand, what would you do? Of course, you'd clean the cut, applying a topical antibacterial cream and bandage the wound to keep it clean while it's healing. So far, so good. But these are *external* treatments. What would you suggest your body do *internally*? Would you think to have your tissues swell to cut off the blood flow to the cut? How about sending special chemicals to the area so the blood will clot? Would you remember to send extra white blood cells to prevent infection?

The fact is, if you had to stop and try to remember all these steps, your hand would fall off before you figured out how to heal it. Fortunately, your Innate Intelligence knows how to heal this kind of wound. It also knows what to do when you get a cold, hurt your back, get a headache or have an allergic reaction.

The purpose of health care should be to allow the body's wisdom to do the healing without interfering with this process. When you use chemicals or surgical procedures at the outset, you interfere with your body's intelligence and interfere with the healing functions before you know if your body's wisdom is adequate to correct the the problem.

Chiropractic philosophy begins with the premise that there is an order to the universe. Nothing is random or meaningless in our world. There is a reason for everything. Granted, we may not always recognize that reason, let alone understand it, but we can be certain that nothing occurs by chance or "just happens."

We know that there is an intelligent order to the universe. A guiding force exists in all living matter, and most definitely in human beings. It's only because of this intelligence that we can continue to exist and operate in this world. Without it, our planet would be a shapeless pile of rocks and debris. Plants wouldn't know how to grow. The animals wouldn't know how to breed and replenish their species. Birds wouldn't know how to fly or fish how to swim.

Now, this premise isn't a matter of blind faith or religious faith on the part of scientists, philosophers and chiropractors. It's based on physical evidence seen in the real world.

Look around you! Can everything in the universe be the result of random selection or luck? Why is a bird's wing perfectly designed for flight, right down to the tiniest pinfeather? Does it just happen that a plant's roots travel downward into the ground and its leaves grow upward? If the universe were really random, at least some plants would send their roots straight up and bury their leaves in the soil. The sun would only come up on random days and it would be difficult to be certain of anything occurring again.

To think the universe is operating without any intelligent plan is like thinking that the Great Sphinx of Egypt was the result of an accidental rock slide!

❄ ❄ ❄

UNIVERSAL INTELLIGENCE

Innate Intelligence is within Universal Intelligence which guides all life. Innate Intelligence is in every living thing. It is revealed when a plant turns its leaves toward the light or when a bird sits on its eggs until they hatch and when a human body knows what to do to heal itself.

Concepts like Universal Intelligence and Innate Intelligence greatly influence your health and your life. Once understood, you'll see why your body always strives to remain healthy. You'll also learn why your body sometimes needs help to function normally and achieve its goal of optimum health and well-being.

"Intelligence is present everywhere in our bodies...our own inner intelligence is far superior to any we can try to substitute from the outside."

Deepak Chopra, M.D.

It requires human intelligence to create a Great Sphinx. Even greater intelligence is needed to create and sustain the natural wonders which surround us. It takes what we call Universal Intelligence. As humans, it's difficult for us to understand what it is, where it comes from or how it works. We know only that it must exist or nothing else would. There are some who equate Universal Intelligence to God. If that makes you comfortable, this theory works as well as any. One thing that is very obvious, through both observation and logic, is that such an Intelligence, by whatever name humans choose to call it, must exist.

For some, this idea is "unscientific." After all, one can't prove it or test it in a research laboratory. Yet, science is now expanding into areas such as quantum physics, and is welcoming fresh ideas. Scientists are even starting to accept the presence of a Universal Intelligence as a basic truth of the universe.

INNATE INTELLIGENCE

"Innate is an individualized portion of the ALL-WISE usually known as spirit."

B.J. Palmer, D.C.

To chiropractors Innate Intelligence is not about how smart someone is—the level of a person's education or his or her ability to learn new material. A person with a Ph.D. in nuclear physics doesn't have any more Innate Intelligence than an aborigine who's never been out of the bush. Innate Intelligence guides us to adapt to our environment in order to survive. It allows nocturnal animals to have eyes that can see in the dark. It makes a leafy plant on a window sill turn its leaves toward the light. Move the plant and it will turn its leaves again. You don't have to tell the plant what to do. The plant knows it has to have light to survive.

Obviously, the plant doesn't use logic to determine that it needs light. A plant doesn't think at all. Yet it knows how to use light, air and water and how to create a new plant. The plant knows what it has to do because it has Innate Intelligence.

Innate Intelligence makes a baby's heart beat, digests food, eliminates waste, uses white blood cells to fight infections, and makes the baby cry when it wants attention. No one has to teach an infant any of these things.

THE TRIUNE OF LIFE

Of course, Innate Intelligence is the basis for proper function, but other factors are required for complete health.

If you were a master carpenter, you would be able to design a piece of furniture, draw out the pattern pieces, cut the wood, assemble the parts, and then stain and wax the finished piece. However, if you didn't have the pencil and paper to draw a pattern, or the tools to cut the wood and put it together, you could not make a cabinet. Or, if you had everything you needed, but lacked the strength to lift the hammer, you could not practice your craft.

Your Innate Intelligence is an expert in building a healthy body. But, if you don't have the proper energy, all the body parts or you are so weak physically and your body is in need of major repair, your body will not reflect health.

In chiropractic, strength is called Energy. The proper set of tools (all your body parts) is called Matter. These three elements, Innate Intelligence, Energy and Matter are known as the *Triune of Life*.

Living beings are like tiny universes. Each one is guided by a personal form of Universal Intelligence (Innate Intelligence) and also, each holds a mini-version of Universal Energy (Innate Energy).

"Chiropractors adjust subluxations, relieving pressure from the nerves so that they can perform their functions in a normal manner. The Innate can and will do the rest."

B.J. Palmer, D.C.

VERTEBRAL SUBLUXATION, OR NERVE INTERFERENCE

If all three elements were always in perfect order, we would be in perfect health. Unfortunately, this is usually not the case.

In our world Innate Matter (our body) doesn't always function at peak performance. The brain sends messages to cells in the body, telling them what they need to do in specific parts of the body. Messages travel along a complex system of nerves. They can run into interference, some of the messengers may take detours, others slow down or lose their way.

Much of this interference occurs along the spine. This is the headquarters of the nerve system. All nerves from the brain travel down this row of interlocking bones, called *Vertebrae*. They branch off and pass through openings along the spine to get to their destinations.

Occasionally, one or more of the vertebrae move out of alignment, we call this *nerve interference*, or a *subluxation(s)*. Where misalignments occur the spinal opening narrows distorting the flow of Innate Energy throughout the body.

"The mysterious breakdowns of the body's intelligence...may be traceable to a single distortion—a wrong detour...

Deepak Chopra, M.D.

If you have nerve interference, your body can't perform efficiently because it isn't getting the right messages from the brain.

Here's an example of what happens. When an unfriendly virus attacks, Innate Intelligence instructs the body to react and fight off the virus. This often means raising the body temperature so the fever can fight off the invader.

If the nerve flow is disturbed because of nerve interference, chemical imbalance occurs and the body will function less efficiently—its ability to fight off an infection is diminished. If you experience one or more of the following symptoms; pain, dizziness, stiffness, weakness, profuse sweating, coughing, diarrhea, fever or stomach upset and vomiting, then it's time to receive an adjustment. Often these conditions are the result of one's body attempting to restore health. Correcting nerve interference will help your body return to normal function.

To adjust the subluxation, then, is to advance mankind, step up his efficiency, increase his ability, make him more natural and more at peace with himself, for all things are possible to him whose body equals his Innate.

B.J. Palmer, D.C.

Jonathan Falman's Experience

My problem began quite unexpectedly. I bent down one day but couldn't stand straight again. At 57, I'm very active. I play a lot of tennis and my job as a mechanic at McDonnell-Douglas requires me to bend and twist in some awkward positions, especially when I have to squeeze through the small openings in some of the jets I work on.

Five days after the problem began, I was still suffering agonizing low back pain. I wasn't able to do anything.

I took the recommendations of several friends and went to see a doctor of chiropractic who took X-rays. I was told that the problem was in my spine; and the doctors explained the spine's direct relation to my general health.

When I came to the chiropractor, I couldn't even reach my knees with my hands. Now I can touch my toes without bending my knees, which I haven't been able to do for more years than I can remember. I can't thank my chiropractor enough.

We chiropractors work with the subtle substance of the soul. We release the prisoned impulses, a tiny rivulet of force, that emanates from the mind and flows over the nerves to the cells and stirs them to life. We deal with the magic power that transforms common food into living, loving, thinking clay; that robes the earth with beauty, and hues and scents the flowers with the glory of the air.

B. J. Palmer

Chapter 3

YOUR MIRACULOUS BODY

The most amazing machine in the history of the natural world is the human body. If you were to purchase this machine it would cost millions of dollars. Once you brought it home you would treat it reverently. However special and valuable, we pay little attention to our body. In this chapter, I want to take you on a short tour of your body and remind you of its spectacular abilities. I want you to think about what would happen if there was interference to the nerve system that controls all body functions.

❊　❊　❊

YOUR DNA—The Mastermind

The movie *Jurassic Park* has certainly illustrated how DNA contains the blueprint for life forms. The author of the novel (from which the movie was made), physician Michael Crichton, speculates that if it were possible to extract the DNA molecules of dinosaurs from amber containing fossilized remains, we could recreate these extinct creatures in today's world. Although it may be nothing more than a hypothetical theory, scientists have recognized the importance of DNA in identifying life forms.

Your body is made up of trillions of cells. Each cell contains DNA (deoxyribonucleic acid). A DNA molecule is so small that it requires an electron microscope to magnify it to be seen. It only takes one two-trillionth of an ounce of DNA to determine the kind of person you will be physically and mentally. In fact, the entire human race could be reproduced by an amount of DNA that would be equivalent to about the size of a dime.

When examined under a microscope, you can see that each DNA molecule contains atoms which are joined together to form a spiral. Unwound they would measure five feet in length! Since each of us begins with one cell, the DNA molecules in this single cell contain all the information needed to build your body. From how you look, to how your body works, all the designs are in your original DNA molecule. Every other cell in your body replicates the original molecule.

Even though there are about five billion people on the earth, each of us has different fingerprints and voiceprints. There are only eight basic fingerprint patterns but no two people have ever been found to have identical prints. Likewise, our voices are all unique. Each of us has a distinct energy wave pattern in our voice which can be charted by scientists. Interestingly enough, this pattern stays the same whether we're shouting or whispering.

As you grow, your cells multiply by dividing over and over again. These cells are so tiny that if you lined up 4,000 of them, the line would only be one inch long. Cells come in many shapes and sizes depending on their function. They take in food and oxygen and eliminate waste. With the exception of brain cells, body cells are replaced by new cells upon completion of their life cycle. About every seven years the cells in the human body have completely been replaced. The reason you can remember things that happened long ago is that you keep your billions of brain cells all your life. They never die off, unless you destroy them.

YOUR BLOOD—The Stream of Life

Your blood is made up of billions of cells. It travels to your veins, arteries and capillaries on a stream of liquid called *plasma*. Innate Intelligence controls this flow of blood. The red cells carry oxygen from your lungs to your tissues. They also take waste gas (carbon dioxide) out of the tissues and carry it back to your lungs where it can be exhaled. A red cell, which lives about four months, makes three thousand trips through your blood stream. About ten million die off each minute but with adequate nourishment new red cells are quickly formed.

Your body is constantly being bombarded by micro-organisms, which often get into the lymph fluid and are carried into the lymph nodes. Once they get there, your white cells, (soldier cells) attack them. On any one day, there can be as many as thirty- to forty-billion soldiers cells protecting you. While these cells are alive they fight off serious infections. Two-thirds of the white cells are made in the marrow of your bones, as are all the red blood cells. They form a clot when you cut yourself, using *fibrin* to

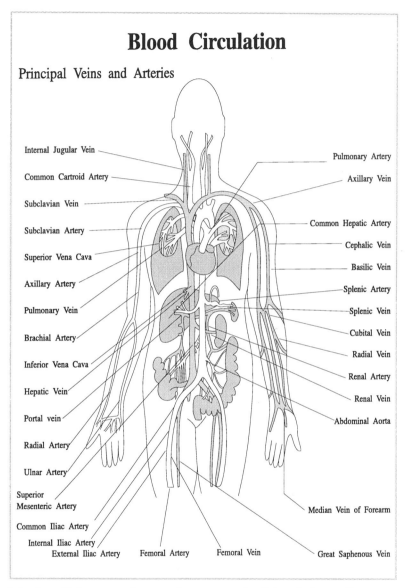

Blood Circulation

Principal Veins and Arteries

Internal Jugular Vein

Common Cartroid Artery

Subclavian Vein

Subclavian Artery

Superior Vena Cava

Axillary Artery

Pulmonary Vein

Brachial Artery

Inferior Vena Cava

Hepatic Vein

Portal vein

Radial Artery

Ulnar Artery

Superior Mesenteric Artery

Common Iliac Artery

Internal Iliac Artery

External Iliac Artery   Femoral Artery   Femoral Vein

Pulmonary Artery

Axillary Vein

Common Hepatic Artery

Cephalic Vein

Basilic Vein

Splenic Artery

Splenic Vein

Cubital Vein

Radial Vein

Renal Artery

Renal Vein

Abdominal Aorta

Median Vein of Forearm

Great Saphenous Vein

block off the opening and prevent the blood from flowing out of your body.

A drop of blood contains about five million red cells and seven thousand white cells, along with thousands of platelets (cells that are not red or white). Blood cells are very small—60 thousand could be put on the head of a pin.

The average adult has four to six quarts of blood —about seven pounds or three-and-a-half quarts of blood for each 100 pounds of body weight. Blood is divided into four primary groups: Type O, which is the most common, Type A, Type B, and Type AB, which is the most rare.

YOUR HEART—The Pump

The heart is the strongest and toughest muscle in your body, weighing from nine to eleven ounces. The average heart beats about 75 times every minute. With each beat, it pumps blood into your lungs to pick up oxygen and out of the lungs to supply the tissues in the body. Both of these actions happen at the same time, even though you only feel one beat. If you could track one blood cell, you would find

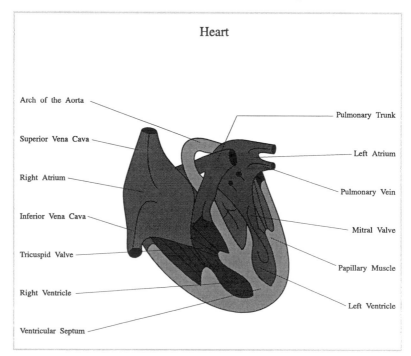

Heart

Arch of the Aorta

Superior Vena Cava

Right Atrium

Inferior Vena Cava

Tricuspid Valve

Right Ventricle

Ventricular Septum

Pulmonary Trunk

Left Atrium

Pulmonary Vein

Mitral Valve

Papillary Muscle

Left Ventricle

it has been pumped throughout your entire circulatory system in sixty minutes. Stretched out end-to-end, our veins and arteries are about 12,000 miles in length, so it requires a strong muscle to pump blood through our bodies.

Normally, your heart pumps about two-and-a-half gallons of blood each minute. When you lie down, your heart slows down and you save about 824 beats each hour you rest. This gives your body more energy to fight disease.

❄ ❄ ❄

YOUR LUNGS—The Bellows

If you have ever seen the way a bellow blows air to fan a fire, you have a pretty good idea of how the lungs work. *Alveoli* or air sacs surround the lungs which are made of a

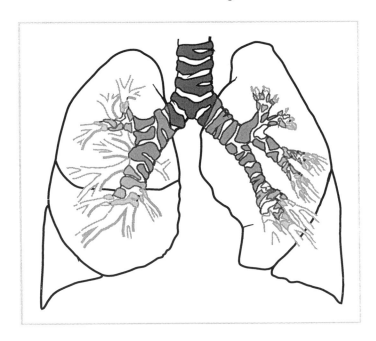

spongy tissue. Bronchial tubes penetrate the lungs, carrying the air you breathe to the single cell air sacs. Blood vessels wind around each sac. The molecules of oxygen leave the air in the sacs and pass into the blood. At the same time, carbon dioxide gas passes from the blood to the air sacs to be exhaled. The whole procedure of exchanging carbon dioxide for oxygen takes less than a second.

In the average twenty-four-hour period, you will use about 90 gallons of pure oxygen or 3000 gallons of air. Your lungs are centered in your chest cavity, protected by your ribs, breast bone and diaphragm, which is a sheet of muscle at the base of your lungs. It's the diaphragm that causes the lungs to expand and contract. As you breathe in, the diaphragm pulls down while your ribs and breast bone moves up. This allows more room for the lungs to expand and fill with air. When you breathe out, the muscles relax and the air is expelled out of your lungs.

❄ ❄ ❄

YOUR RESPIRATORY SYSTEM—The Filter

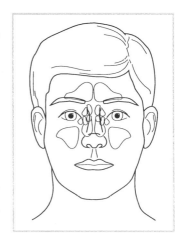

You wouldn't live very long if air went directly into the lungs without being filtered. Your lungs would fill up with dust, pollen, soot, spores, fibers and thousands of other particles floating in the air.

When you breathe, air enters your nose and passes through

your windpipe into your lungs. The nasal passages are lined with a mucus membrane which is moist and covered with tiny hairs called *cilia*. The hairs and mucus trap dirt and germs and keep them from entering your lungs. Your voice box, windpipe and the thousands of small tubes in your lungs are also covered with cilia. These continuously sweep away germs. Coughing and sneezing are Innate safety devices to remove particles from your larynx and nasal passages.

The mucus in your nose carries a germicide called *lysozyme*. This same germ-killing substance is found in your tears, and moves from your tear ducts into your nose to moisten and protect the nasal tissues.

"Innate knows more in one second than you can ever know."

B.J. Palmer, D.C.

YOUR MUSCLES—Doing the Work

Each muscle consists of long, thin cells wrapped in bundles and held together by a tissue covering called the *fascia*. Some muscles are connected to tendons, which are strong white cords that anchor muscles to the bones. More than six-hundred muscles reside in your body, enabling you to perform even the simplest act.

There are three kinds of muscles. The *Voluntary* muscles move when you cause them to. These are the muscles that you use to raise your arm or walk or turn your head. The *smooth* muscles operate without any conscious input from you. These include the muscles in the stomach, intestine and bladder. The heart is a muscle, too. It's made up of cells that look like tiny planks and it has more power than any other muscle in the body.

Muscles get their energy from oxygen, sugars and fat. They keep you warm by emitting heat. Muscles need activity. If you don't do something physical every day, your muscles can atrophy, and your general health will decline.

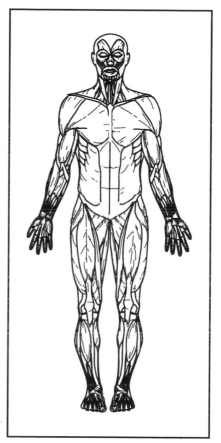

YOUR BRAIN — A Human Computer

The human brain has the potential to be faster and store more information than any computer ever developed. Unfortunately, we have only learned to use a tiny percentage of our brain's capacity. Even so, your brain receives and interprets thousands of signals from every nerve in your body during every second of the day. The largest part of the brain, the *cerebrum*, relays messages from the sensory organs, such as the nose, eyes, ears, tongue and skin, to the various parts of your body. Certain areas of the cerebrum are responsible for specific functions, such as memory, reading comprehension, physical movement and so on. Another part of the brain, the *medulla oblongata*, controls automatic processes like breathing and keeping your heart beating. The *cerebellum*, is responsible for

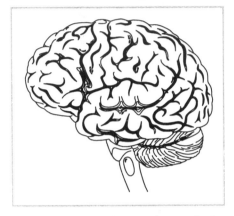

balance and motor coordination.

Your brain is connected to all parts of the body. The tail of the brain—the spinal cord emerges through an opening in the skull called the Foramen Magnum (a large hole). The spinal cord goes through the twenty-four bony rings or vertebrae and the spinal nerves branch out from the various vertebrae to carry information to and from every part of the body. As stated before, when the nerves are impeded because the vertebrae are out of alignment, the result is a lack of normal function.

❄ ❄ ❄

YOUR STOMACH—The Food Processor

Your stomach has amazing power. It can produce hydrochloric acid to break down the food you eat—an acid so strong that if put on your hand, blisters would appear. Hydrochloric acid produces *pepsin* and *renin*, two other chemicals that prepare food to be digested by the intestines. The lining of the stomach is made of cells that produce tiny flakes of mucus. These line and protect the stomach just like shingles protect the roof of a house.

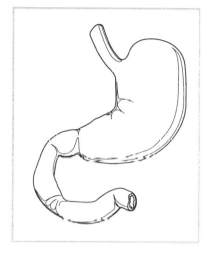

Two-and-a-half quarts of gastric juices produced by your stomach each day allow you to digest a meal in one to seven hours, depending on what you have eaten. When the stomach is full, it contracts, helping to break down the food and push it towards the lower end of the stomach, the *pylorus*. From there, it goes into the intestines where all the nutrients are removed for use by the body and the waste is carried out of the body.

If you exercise immediately after you eat, or if you are very upset, you will slow down the digestive process and feel nauseated. Lack of food causes the stomach to contract in a rhythmic pattern and we identify this as hunger pains.

YOUR SKIN—The Largest Organ of All

Although skin is only 1/16th to 1/8th inch thick, it has very important functions. The surface of the skin is called the *epidermis* and the layer below it is called the *dermis*. It is the epidermis that usually gets scraped when we skin a knee and unless we cut the dermis, we don't bleed. The lower layers of the epidermis contain a pigment called *melanin* which determines the skin color. The more melanin

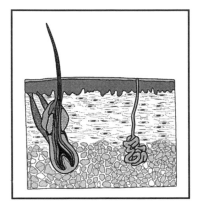

you have, the darker your skin.

Your skin contains sweat and oil glands. Two million sweat glands allow you to excrete liquid waste material and stay cool through perspiration. The oil glands serve to waterproof your skin while keeping it from becoming too dry. The oil glands also keep your hair smooth and shiny.

Blood circulates through your skin, helping to regulate body heat. If you get too hot, the blood vessels in your skin expand coming closer to the surface of the skin where, the outside air cools it. When you are cold, the blood vessels contract, so less blood is near the skin's surface.

(NOTE: Exercise pushes blood near the surface of the skin. Fright moves it away.)

The *papillae* contains the nerves which connect the epidermis to the dermis and enable us to experience the sensation of touch.

Our skin doesn't wear away because new cells constantly renew the surface of the epidermis and the old cells die and flake away.

❄ ❄ ❄

YOUR HANDS—The All-Purpose Tools

Have you ever taken the time to think about all the things you do with your hands? These really are remarkable tools that can distinguish size, shape, texture and temperature. They move, grasp or release objects, hold a pen to write, or play a piano or stitch a fine seam.

The millions of tiny nerve endings send touch impulses to the brain which convert sensations into reactions and perceptions. Just by touching a stove with your hand, your brain knows it is smooth and metallic, cool to the touch in some places and hot in others. It also knows that as your hand gets closer to the heat, you need to be careful you don't get burned.

The movements of your fingers are controlled by tendons—strong fibers that operate like a pulley cord to make the bones and muscles do what you want them to. The coordination between the tendons, muscles and bones is so perfect we're not even aware of it.

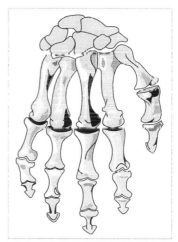

There are fifty-four bones in your hand, the thumb bone is the most versatile and the strongest. We tend to take our hands for granted, however, if deprived of the use of our hands, we'd quickly realize how vital they are to everything we do.

❋ ❋ ❋

YOUR FEET—Engineering Marvels

One fourth of your body's bones are in your feet. Each foot contains twenty-six bones, linked together with thirty-three joints and attached by ligaments. The arch in your foot is

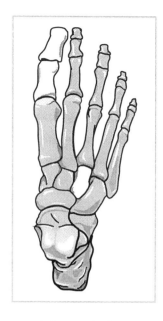

an engineering marvel, built to withstand several hundred times its own weight and still keep the body balanced with mathematical precision. Five *metatarsal* bones are in each arch. They are attached to the *phalanges* or toe bones at one end and the *tarsals* at the other. The tarsals connect the foot to the leg.

The arch distributes your weight evenly over your foot. If you weigh ninety-six pounds, the metatarsal bones attached to your big toes support eighty-eight pounds of the weight and those attached to the smaller toes support the remaining eight pounds.

The average person walks about 30,000 steps—twelve miles each day. At ninety-six pounds, you put 2,880,000 pounds of pressure on your feet in any twenty-four-hour period. And that's just walking! If you run, each step adds ten times your weight to your feet.

Because your feet are below your heart, the blood has to flow up from your feet against gravity. Inside your veins there are tiny gate valves which allow the blood to travel upward preventing it from flowing back down and collecting in your feet.

(NOTE: When you experience an emotion like fear, the blood rushes to your brain and the temperature in your feet goes down. This is why we say someone "has cold feet" when they are afraid.)

The feet, like other parts of the body are truly amazing

and wonderful mechanisms. It seems only Innate Intelligence could create such a remarkable living machine.

❄ ❄ ❄

YOUR CHEMISTRY LAB—Your "24-Hour Drugstore"

"Medical men have searched the world for remedies, desiring an antidote. Chiropractors find the cause in the person ailing."

B.J. Palmer, D.C.

Your magical chemistry lab supplies you with hundreds of chemicals to keep your body functioning properly. Chemicals keep your sinuses clear and your eyes working well, chemicals raise and lower your blood pressure and your body temperature, chemicals control your moods and help you digest your food and eliminate waste. There are also chemicals which guarantee your reproductive organs will work. Your body also produces insulin and cortisone and adrenaline and antibiotics to fight infection—and this is only a fraction of the list. Science has much more to learn about the chemicals your body continually manufactures to keep you healthy.

Your magical chemistry lab includes specific instructions about how much of a chemical you need at any moment. It releases enough digestive juices to dissolve your stomach contents after a meal and enough insulin to deal with the sugar you had in that piece of pie. If you're frightened, it will give you a shot of adrenaline to give you

51

an extra boost of energy to take action. It releases clotting chemicals to the site of a wound and relaxants to allow you to get a good night's rest.

Your "laboratory" supplies everything to you at no cost. All it requires is that you give yourself the good care you deserve.

Your body is the most superb chemistry lab ever devised. It's as if you had the world's smartest health professional living inside you. Luckily our bodies work without any help from us. In fact, they work in spite of the mistreatment we often heap upon them.

Our Innate Intelligence controls every biological, chemical and physical action and reaction. When your Innate Intelligence is allowed to fully express itself, you have a better chance of reaching your maximum health potential. If you are functioning normally, every chemical you need will be delivered when it's needed, in the exact amount, twenty-four hours a day. It's a remarkably efficient system.

❊　❊　❊

LACK OF PROPER CHEMICALS—Chaos

Timely delivery of chemicals to different areas of the body goes unnoticed but if delayed or canceled, the effect is often dramatic.

For instance, you can't hold a pen to write unless your brain produces a chemical called *dopamine* which stimulates the basal ganglia and keeps your extremities from shaking. A person with Parkinson syndrome is missing dopamine and can't thread a needle or hold a paper without shaking uncontrollably.

Chemicals ingested into the body often interfere with its natural action. For instance, you have a natural sleep cycle because your body produces the proper chemicals to allow you to sleep. However, if you drink a cup of coffee just before bedtime, the caffeine in the coffee may interfere with the chemical balance and sleep may elude you.

Sugar is a chemical that has adverse affects on the body—throwing it off balance. The famed pediatrician Lendon Smith, M.D., was asked to study a group of children who were considered hyperkinetic or hyperactive. He found they were routinely given the drug Ritalin to calm them down but they turned into little zombies. However, after eating a heavily sugared meal they would again become very active.

Dr. Smith showed that the children's hyperkinetic behavior could be reversed by altering their diet and eliminating all the sugared breakfast cereals, lunch time cake, mid-afternoon ice cream and before bedtime candy. Once children's sugar levels were brought under control, each child's pancreas didn't work overtime to produce enough insulin and the result for all was a normal blood sugar level and modified behavior.

Your body doesn't want or need sugar. The body's chemistry lab isn't prepared to cope with it. And the result is all the unpleasant symptoms of high blood sugar hyperactivity or low blood sugar lethargy and depression.

Alcohol is another chemical that negatively affects our body. It creates, a chemical imbalance in the brain and often people's behavior. Observe people who have had too many cocktails at a party. One person might be belligerent and hostile. Someone else might become loud and obnoxious, while another might become emotional and cry or just fall into a stupor.

What we consider "normal" behavior is the result of chemical balance, which comes from well-functioning glands producing the chemicals at the command of the brain and spinal cord. The glands have a better chance of making the body function normally when there is no interference.

Nerve interference can bring all this "chemical laboratory" activity to a halt. Without any recognizable symptoms, your body's nerve supply may be interfered with causing your good health to change, depriving your body of the naturally produced chemicals to function properly, lowering your resistance and weakening your immune system.

Invest in your health, take time for regular check-ups. It's the best gift you can give yourself and your family.

> **The more you understand the way your body functions the more you will be motivated to take care of yourself. Doctors of Chiropractic are primarily interested in the proper function of body tissue and organs of the body—all controlled by the nerve system.**

Chapter 4

VISITING A CHIROPRACTOR

Nerve interference has become a silent epidemic. Schedule a regular spinal checkup the way you schedule a routine dental check-up or a periodic eye exam. How long has it been since your spine was examined? For many people a scoliosis check in junior high was their last spinal examination.

When a chiropractor sees a new patient, it's common to find that muscles, ligaments, nerves, and internal organs are not in perfect order. The spine, too, often experiences some kind of degeneration.

❄ ❄ ❄

THE PHYSICAL EXAMINATION

Your first visit will consist of a consultation and complete spinal examination. Most doctors will also provide some education if you are not familiar with chiropractic care.

"Chiropractors adjust the cause of dis-ease instead of treating the effects."

B.J. Palmer, D.C.

The first thing you'll be asked to do when you visit a chiropractic office is fill out forms regarding personal information and health history. Then, the doctor will have a consultation with you and give you a chiropractic examination.

The most common examination is called palpation. The doctor carefully feels—or palpates—the entire spinal region to detect nerve interference. Other methods or instruments may be used to verify the findings. All of the examination techniques used by chiropractors are safe, painless and non-invasive.

Indications of nerve interference show up on an X-ray, soft tissue damage to nerves, muscles or discs—nerve impingement—can't be seen. For further diagnosis, some chiropractors utilize imaging tools such as MRI's, Thermography and Paraspinal EMGs and CT (CAT) scans. Your chiropractor will explain these methods in greater detail.

Use of X-rays should be a concern, but keep in mind that chiropractic does not use radiation as treatment or therapy but only as a diagnostic tool. Chiropractic radiology generally exposes patients to a lot less radiation than similar orthopedic and medical examinations. Screens, shields and high-speed X-ray film further reduce the danger of over exposure.

Chiropractors believe that the benefit must always justify the risks that are inherent. That's why we talk to our patients honestly, explain the risks and answer questions in non-technical terms.

❄ ❄ ❄

REPORT OF FINDINGS

After testing and diagnosis, you'll receive a report of the doctor's findings. You'll be told if there is any nerve interference and how severe it is.

You and your doctor will discuss the health of your spine and the doctor will outline a course of care needed to correct the nerve interference. This may include spinal adjustments, beneficial exercise and changes to your life-style.

Chiropractors don't treat symptoms. Our job is to locate the cause of dis-ease, the nerve interference, and correct it. Frequent adjustments may be required at the beginning.

As your condition improves, the number of adjustments will decrease and you'll be placed on wellness care. Don't expect nerve interference to be corrected in a few visits. It will take continued adjusting to be certain the vertebrae have returned to their proper position and your muscles and ligaments can continue to hold them firmly in place.

Once you are properly "back together," your doctor will perform periodic spinal checks to make sure your spine remains free of nerve interference.

There are three levels of chiropractic care. First, is an Intensive Care Phase, Level I. During this time, the chiropractor's objective is to reduce stress damage to the spine and nervous system.

You might be in a situation where you have pain, or disease that has convinced you to seek help. Realize that the chiropractic adjustments are helping you immediately but you have to understand healing takes time. Your condition didn't occur overnight. Be willing to change your personal habits and follow the doctor's advice to move the process along.

During the Level I period, you may be seeing your D.C. every day—or at least three times a week depending on the need.

Level II is the Reconstructive Phase. Now, the spine is nearly or completely aligned but it has to be monitored while it becomes stronger and holds the adjustment for longer periods of time. This stage is critical. Complete correction cannot take place if you don't have your spine checked regularly to be very sure there isn't a reoccurrence of nerve interference. During Level II, you may be seeing your chiropractor from one to two times a week.

Level III is the Wellness Phase. Now, your spine is holding its adjustment. This phase is similar to having your eyes checked or having your teeth cleaned. You want to visit your chiropractor on a regular basis. In this way, you can detect and correct nerve interference early and enhance your body's Innate ability to express its maximum health potential.

❋ ❋ ❋

PATIENT EDUCATION PROGRAMS

Unlike many other doctors, chiropractors don't work ON our patients. We work WITH them. Health care and wellness care become a joint project for both the doctor and patient. To help educate the patients, most doctors offer some kind of information or educational program for new patients. This might consist of reading material, video tapes, a workshop, or orientation program.

If your D.C. offers a patient education program, take advantage of it. Read the material you receive. Watch the video tapes or listen to the audio tapes. Attend the presentations. Ask questions! The more you know and understand about chiropractic, the better able you'll be to help yourself.

Remember to visit your chiropractor even when you're under the care of a medical doctor. Doctors in other disciplines can't determine if you have nerve interference, they haven't been trained to recognize it. Your D.C. may help your body correct a condition naturally that an M.D. would treat with artificial chemicals or surgery.

"It is useless to administer a powder, potion, or pill to the stomach when the body needs an adjustment."

B.J. Palmer, D.C.

PUT YOUR MIND AT REST

In 1994, the American Heart Association (AHA) generated a great deal of publicity by announcing that researchers at the Stanford University School of Medicine had surveyed 486 California neurologists about the number of patients they had treated in the preceding two years. Specifically, the researchers wanted to know about those patients who

59

had suffered a stroke within 24 hours of cervical manipulation.

According to the AHA, the study showed that there was a "small but significant risk" of a stroke occurring within twenty-four hours after cervical manipulation. The newspapers took the story and ran with it. Within days, headlines declared that *"Stroke Can Be Triggered by Twist of Neck, Study Claims."*

In every medium, the story was reported with sensationalism. It was so slanted that chiropractors were put in the worst light imaginable—as if chiropractic and strokes were almost synonymous.

If that's what you read and heard—here's the truth.

◆ While 486 neurologists were questioned, (all of whom are in direct competition with chiropractors) only 177 physicians responded and of those, only 37 claimed they had seen cases in which there might be a connection between cervical manipulation and the onset of a stroke.

◆ The study was a small one, never published, and not considered significant even by the researchers who set it up. Dr. Gregory W. Albers was one of the Stanford researchers. He said that the study "...was a small survey with a small sample size and it wasn't anything to make a big fuss over." He told me: "There's no question that probably most medical procedures carry a much greater risk — and there's no question what the leading causes of strokes are and its not chiropractic."

◆ Dr. Carlini said "...almost all interventions by allopathic physicians have a higher complication rate than chiropractic."

◆ As the benefits of chiropractic adjustments gain credibility there are an increasing number of M.D.s, Physical Therapists (PTs), etc. who are attempting to train themselves in manipulation techniques at weekend seminars. This type of inadequate training presents a very real danger to the publics health, safety and welfare.

◆ Manipulation: "the forceful passive movement of a joint beyond its active limit of motion. It does not imply the use of precision, specificity, or the correction of nerve interference and, therefore, is not synonymous with the chiropractic adjustment."

◆ Adjustment: "the adjustment is the specific application of forces to facilitate the body's correction of nerve interference."

What we have is an all-too-common *leap of faith* by the media regarding an AHA article or study. Indeed, there has been the extremely rare occurrence of stroke following a cervical manipulation but statistics show one stroke per several million. In any procedure, there is an element of risk because of the individual history of the patient, but statistically, your chance of dying from a bee sting or being killed by lightning is more likely. Many of the stories I have heard have been hearsay and rumor and have exploited the very rare occurrence of a stroke. You can be confident when you walk out of your chiropractors office, after receiving an adjustment your overall health will be improved, not threatened.

Andrew Sanderson's Experience

About thirty years ago, I had a football injury. Over the next several years, I began to have pain in my left knee, a constant dull ache in the lower back on the right side and sinus trouble. I went to my medical doctors for help and they said I would have to live with this the rest of my life. The diagnosis was a permanently damaged nerve. The physicians suggested corrective surgery.

I became very depressed. I couldn't sleep at night and I was very difficult to live with. I was going through hell and so was my family. It was then that I was convinced to try chiropractic. After my first few visits to my chiropractor, I felt a great deal of relief. Now I feel like a new person. My back is greatly improved, without surgery, and it seems as if I never even had knee problems or sinus trouble. It changed my life. When you feel good, you look good and you develop a healthy attitude. It wasn't very long before everyone noticed the great improvement in me. My only regret is that I waited so long!

Doctors of Chiropractic are committed to patient education. Patients appreciate knowing in advance the value and purpose of every procedure before it is rendered. Ask questions! Get involved!

Chapter 5

HERE'S TO YOUR HEALTH

I've discussed the body's ability to heal itself—the army of white blood cells, antibodies, leukocytes, mast cells, neutrophils and eosinophils are internal antibiotic soldiers which patrol and protect every inch of the body from injury and infection.

Even when the body organism is hosting a serious condition, we still have the capacity to heal a cut or overcome an infection.

Medical journals constantly print stories of patients who have recovered spontaneously from incurable illness. Patients who have been given six months to live, are still telling the story thirty years later. There's no definite answer to why this happens. No one understands spontaneous remission but all health care professionals acknowledge that we carry within us a miraculous ability to heal ourselves.

Given our body's ability to heal itself, why do we get sick? Why don't we heal ourselves every time? There are genetic factors we don't understand that strongly affect how our Innate Wisdom works to heal us. It's the mission of every chiropractor to help patients raise their natural and Innate healing ability to its highest potential.

Chiropractic's main concern is not with the trauma that follows accidents, most of which is emergency first aid—setting bones, stitching wounds closed, and removing foreign objects. That is your medical doctor's job. This is an example of how two divergent healthcare philosophies can compliment each other and forge a cooperative effort.

Unfortunately, other problems are often handled with drugs. These dangerous, artificial chemicals are dispensed to control the symptoms—lower the fever, kill germs and deaden pain. Instead of correcting the underlying cause, these warning signals are ignored, and healing is actually delayed. Our society is full of people who are little more than walking medicine cabinets. They take handfuls of pills throughout the day. Instead of finding out and correcting what is causing their high blood pressure, they take medicine to lower it. Instead of determining the underlying metabolic reason for their condition, they rely on artificial chemicals for a temporary cover-up. If they stop taking the medicine, the condition returns. This isn't health and healing. This is containment and control.

As a chiropractor, I believe that at the root of many of these conditions is nerve interference. This isn't to say that if your spine is healthy, you'll never have a sick day and you'll live forever. No one can promise you that. We come into the world marked "terminal" because as human beings we all die. However, without nerve interference, you can be confident you have a better chance for a longer, healthier existence.

✢ ✢ ✢

THE NEUROLOGICAL BASIS OF DISEASE

If you are still unclear about the connection between the spine and overall health, you need to know the story of Masha and Dasha Krivoshlyapova, one of the most unusual sets of co-joined twins ever born. When they were born, on January 4, 1950, their mother was told they had died shortly after birth. In fact, they had been taken to a Soviet institution near Moscow for study, observation and experimentation. For nearly forty years, they were isolated from their family and the world.

Co-joined (Siamese) twins result when a single fertilized egg doesn't split completely, as it does in the case of identical twins. Instead the egg remains joined at some point and the children are born partially attached. Usually, these children are spontaneously aborted as embryos, but on rare occasions, they are born alive. If the connection isn't extensive, they can sometimes be separated successfully. In a 1993 case, one twin was sacrificed so her sister, the stronger of the two, could have a chance to live.

In the case of Masha and Dasha, the co-joining was so extensive that an operation to separate them would have killed them both. It was the unique way in which they were joined that caused the Soviet scientists to be so interested in them.

The girls were born with four arms and three legs. They stood on two legs, one controlled by each twin and a vestigial third leg remained in the air behind them. It's not surprising that it took them until they were five before they developed the coordination to be able to walk.

65

Their upper intestines were separate but they shared a lower intestine and rectum. They had four kidneys and one bladder and one reproductive system. From the waist up, they were two distinct persons with interconnected circulatory systems, so they shared each other's blood. When a virus entered one sister's bloodstream, it soon appeared in the other sister's blood as well. However, illness affected them quite differently. In fact, in an interview in 1989, Masha complained they had always been treated as one person when their medical files were quite diverse.

For instance, Dasha was near-sighted, caught cold easily and was right-handed. Masha, who was left-handed, smoked occasionally but still had a stronger constitution than her sister, even though she had slightly higher blood pressure.

The question that puzzled scientists was why one sister would get measles and the other wouldn't, even though the germ was in both bodies. Russian pathologist, A. D. Speransky, realized that the nerve system had a definite role in the development of disease. The healthier the nerve system, the more the body could fight off illness. In the case of Masha and Dasha, what was it that caused one to be sick and the other to stay well?

The answer became apparent. While they shared their circulatory, digestive, excretory, lymphatic, and endocrine system and had a common skeletal system from where they were joined at the hips, they had separate spinal columns and skulls. Thus they had separate spinal cords and separate brains. This was the only significant difference between them!

These remarkable twins lived their lives as a walking

laboratory in which scientists verified that disease and sickness do indeed have a neurological basis. Because of them, researchers have proved one can't get sick simply from being exposed to germs. One's body has to supply those germs with a fertile breeding ground where they can multiply and grow. That's why one twin could be ill when the other wasn't.

Each of us breathes in millions of germs every time we inhale and we breathe out even more germs when we exhale. If the cause of illness were as simple as being exposed to bacteria, we would all be sick all the time.

One last note about Masha and Dasha. In 1989, they were released from the institution, rejoined their mother and were looking forward to a happier future. However, as distressing as the first forty years of their lives were, they could take some comfort in the knowledge that they have significantly advanced our understanding of how the brain and spine affect our general health.

❄ ❄ ❄

THE ADJUSTMENT

At the heart of chiropractic care is the adjustment. A spinal adjustment is a specific application of forces used to facilitate the body's correction of nerve interference. The force must be given with the right amount of pressure in the proper direction at the right time. While it is usually done with the doctors hands, adjusting instruments are used too.

We often hear that patients believe there are different adjustments for different conditions. They think there is a specific adjustment for high blood pressure that is different from the adjustment for a headache. The adjustment has one purpose and one purpose only—to correct or reduce nerve interference. The potential healing of a symptomatic condition or disease often results from the correct nerve flow to the affected area and improvement of your overall body chemistry. Remember, the symptom is usually the warning signal to alert you that something is wrong.

If you don't have any symptoms and visit your chiropractor as part of a wellness program, you won't receive an adjustment unless you have nerve interference. Having a disease or other health condition won't warrant an adjustment unless you have nerve interference.

"In the future, chiropractic will be valued for its preventative qualities as much as for relieving and adjusting the cause of ailments."

B.J. Palmer, D.C.

What you can expect from your adjustment is a feeling of peace and relaxation that can last from a day to a week. Patients often comment that they experience a better night's sleep and increased energy. It's common to hear that they went home and tackled that project they've been putting off for months.

Some patients report that their symptoms start to go away after the first adjustment, while others don't feel any immediate difference. If you don't feel a change, don't be discouraged. Often you are not aware of internal improvements.

Some patients may feel discomfort after their first adjustment, ranging from a headache to just general fatigue. In almost every case, this feeling goes away within the next couple adjustments.

This discomfort is often due to a detoxification of the body after adjustments. As poisons leave the system, they could create a headache or slight head cold, even a slight fever and a feeling of lethargy.

Muscles may become sore after being adjusted. You may feel sore like you had a workout at the gym. This condition is always temporary and disappears as your muscles gain strength and flexibility.

Spinal nerves that have been impinged and stressed for many years are suddenly coming back to life. These changes are exciting! As they heal, they become sensitive and the old injury pains may return during a necessary and beneficial body phenomenon called "retracing." During "retracing," the healing process is repeated as if the injury had happened yesterday instead of possibly years before.

If your response to an adjustment is euphoria, it's most likely because the newly freed nerves are sending Innate Energy through the opened passages and releasing the physical stress you've become accustomed to feeling. Life is being turned on.

If you feel little change, it may be that your general health is very good—the nerve interference was caught at an early stage before much damage occurred. Each of us is different and no two of us react the same. But everyone will benefit from the correction of nerve interference.

❄ ❄ ❄

RETRACING

Chiropractors have found that body tissues have a memory

which records and holds on to the traumas, injuries and accidents it has experienced. Along with the memory of physical pain, the body also recalls the feelings of fright, shock, or anger and hysteria that accompanied the trauma. When the patient begins healing after an adjustment, it is possible to re-experience some discomfort from an old injury. If this happens, patience is needed to work it through.

Although, retracing is often low key and almost unnoticeable, it can be dramatic for a short time. When it is intense, the patients may feel worse instead of better. Unfortunately, if the patient isn't prepared for this reaction, he or she may terminate the care and cheat themselves out of recovery.

The idea of retracing is used in several branches of healing. John Upledger, Doctor of Osteopathy, calls retracing *unwinding*. Homeopathy refers to it as *flashbacks* and states that according to the three part healing process called Hering's Law, cures occur first, from the inside to the exterior; second, from the most vital to the least vital; and third, in reverse order from how the symptoms appeared.

Psychologists recommend *re-scripting* in order to come to terms with unpleasant past experiences. Re-scripting involves working through past history and rewriting it to have the outcome you wanted.

Typical examples of retracing which occur on the path to healing might be the return of original symptomatic pain after several adjustments. While the pain can be severe, it usually clears up quickly.

These are further examples of how our body strives to heal itself in ways we don't fully understand.

TIME TO HEAL

One of the first questions many chiropractic patients ask is: How long is this going to take? This is a question they may not think to ask a medical doctor. Some drug treatments are prescribed for a lifetime. The chiropractor cannot be expected to undo years of dis-ease in a single visit. It just doesn't work that way.

Your doctor will try to tell you how long it might take before you achieve maximum correction. Whatever the answer, it will be based on three considerations.

First, the doctor will look at the objective results of any diagnostic instrumentation or tests and your physical examination. Second, the doctor will assess the experience with other patients who had similar nerve interference patterns. Third, he or she will consider those characteristics that are unique to you, including your age, how long you've had your nerve interference, your general health history, genetic factors, emotional stress and diet.

The secret is to be patient. Work with your doctor and be very honest about how you feel about your care. The better your relationship with your chiropractor, the better your total healing experience.

"Why search the world over for an exterminator or an antidote for dis-ease? Why not look for the cause of the ailments in the person affected and then correct it?"

B.J. Palmer, D.C.

❄ ❄ ❄

"I'D RATHER DO IT MYSELF!"

Have you ever bent over and heard your spine snap, crackle and pop like a bowl of breakfast cereal? Have you ever gotten out of bed in the morning and moved in exaggerated gestures to make your body create popping sounds, after which you felt immeasurably better for awhile? Have you ever thought you didn't need to see a chiropractor because you could do an adjustment on yourself?

Every doctor has, at one time or another, been at a social function where someone wants to demonstrate how easy it is to "crack" themselves. They proceed to assume a variety of positions that cause large popping sounds to emanate from their spine. "See," they say triumphantly, "how hard is it to do that?"

The truth is, the more you can stretch your spine, the healthier your spine will be. Spinal exercises or stretches, like yoga, are good for you and will probably make you feel better. However, if the vertebrae aren't moving when your spine is "popping" from these stretches, they will continue to make cracking sounds until your doctor has been able to adjust the cause of your nerve interference and correct it. Only your chiropractor knows the exact technique and force necessary to correct your nerve interference.

It's also possible that you have a misalignment which is beneficial. Sometimes, the body has to misalign the vertebrae in order to prop up a weakened area of the spine. These are called compensatory or defensive misalignments. The doctor of chiropractic will recognize that and not attempt to change it. It takes expertise to determine the difference between compensatory misalignment and nerve interference. If you or a well meaning friend play around with spinal manipulation, you can do real harm if you further weaken an area that's already in trouble.

One other word of caution. Occasionally we hear of someone who was paralyzed, and after falling out of a wheelchair, suddenly could walk. It's true that in rare instances there is an accidental adjustment that restores mobility to people who have been afflicted with limited mobility for months or years. However, these instances are so rare that they are usually well publicized when they occur. When it happens, it's magical. But don't assume it's going to happen to you. Statistically, you'd have a better chance of winning the lottery. Instead, call a chiropractor and have your spine checked out so you can be your best every day.

"While other professions are concerned with changing the environment to suit the weakened body, chiropractic is concerned with strengthening the body to suit the environment."

B.J. Palmer, D.C.

Everyday scientists and researchers are proving what doctors of chiropractic have known since 1895.

Chapter 6

A CHIROPRACTOR'S EDUCATION

Two years after discovering the benefit of chiropractic care, D.D. Palmer opened the first chiropractic college. It was 1897 in Davenport, Iowa, when the Palmer Infirmary and Chiropractic Institute opened its doors. Less than a century later, there are eighteen chiropractic colleges in the United States and eight in six foreign countries.

Chiropractic education is every bit as comprehensive as is medical education. Before being accepted by a chiropractic college, students must have completed a minimum of two years of undergraduate work with a heavy emphasis on basic sciences.

Once in chiropractic college, the four-year course of study is longer than that required of most medical students. In addition to classroom and lab work, each student chiropractor must complete a period of internship during which students care for patients under the close supervision of instructors. This is often followed by an *ex*-ternship program during which students assist field chiropractors in their offices. Since these students don't yet have degrees and licenses, they don't adjust spines. They are there to assist, observe and learn.

CHIROPRACTIC COMPARED TO MEDICAL EDUCATION		
	CHIROPRACTIC Classroom Hours	MEDICAL Classroom Hours
Anatomy	540	508
Physiology	240	326
Pathology	360	401
Chemistry	165	325
Microbiology	120	114
Diagnosis	630	324
Neurology	320	112
X-Ray	360	148
Psychiatry	60	144
Obstetrics	60	148
Orthopedics	210	156
Total Hours	3,065	2,706

This comparison chart is based on the review of curriculum catalogues from eleven chiropractic colleges and twenty-two medical schools in the United States. It clearly shows that chiropractors are among the best trained health practitioners you can find. Please note that chiropractic schools study both geriatrics and pediatrics, while eye, ear, nose, throat and dermatology are combined with diagnosis.

After students have acquired the necessary foundation

of knowledge during the early part of their schooling, they later focus on specialized subjects, including chiropractic philosophy and practice, along with chiropractic diagnosis and adjusting techniques that aren't taught in any other health care field.

Before obtaining their degrees, all students must complete approximately nine-hundred hours of work in the clinic setting. Because chiropractic students don't have to spend time studying pharmacology or surgery, as their medical counterparts do, they are given additional training in anatomy, nutrition, diagnosis, palpation, X-ray and a variety of adjusting techniques. In fact, chiropractic students log more educational hours in these subjects than their medical counterparts.

After new chiropractors have graduated, they must then pass a state license exam in any state where they wish to practice. Most graduates take the National Board of Chiropractic Examination which tests the doctors' knowledge in many areas. These particular tests are so comprehensive that most states now accept them as the state licence exam. In addition, a Doctor of Chiropractic must also pass a practical exam and interview conducted by the State Board of Chiropractic Examiners in the state where they are seeking a license.

Cause and Cure

"A cause must be adjusted, corrected, fixed. To cure, you must treat effects, apply something to the results. There in lies the greatest transforming value of chiropractic; it adjusts causes, but does not treat effects."

B.J. Palmer, D.C.

❊ ❊ ❊

Eleanor Drusart's Experience

I first injured my back 20 years ago and I've been having back trouble off and on ever since. The last four years I'd been having muscle spasms in my back which became more frequent and progressively worse. I had constant headaches and was irritable, nervous, tired and depressed, and I had not had my period for the last four years. An orthopedic doctor I had been seeing recommended surgery but couldn't guarantee it would help.

Because I'm a nurse, I rejected the idea of going to a chiropractor. Instead, I just suffered, spending several days in bed with pain killers, a taped-up back and a heating pad. Finally, I was in constant pain and couldn't take it any more. One day several friends told me of the help they'd received from their chiropractor, so I made an appointment to see him that very day. That's when I had my miracle.

After my first adjustment, I left the office and got in my car to leave. Without any warning I started my menstrual cycle. This may sound incredible but that's what happened. I no longer have any muscle spasms or back pain. I'm doing things I haven't done in years. I don't take pain killers or tranquilizers since I started my adjustments. I really enjoy living again! I hope someday chiropractors work as an integral part of the medical profession.

Chapter 7

YOUR CHILD & CHIROPRACTIC

Every baby needs to have a healthy spinal column. It's the framework that will support your child throughout his or her growing years and adulthood. Studies have shown that newborn infants often enter the world with spinal trauma due to the birth process. Even under the best conditions, birthing can be difficult for the infant who has spent nine months cradled in the dark, warm "waterbed" of the womb. It's very important to have your infant checked by a chiropractor shortly after his or her birth to be certain that there isn't any nerve interference. Periodic checks should continue throughout your child's lifetime.

Robert S. Mendelsohn, M.D., was one of America's leading pediatricians and a vocal proponent of home delivery. In his consciousness-raising book, *Confessions of a Medical Heretic*, he discussed how babies born in the hospital are six times more likely to suffer distress during labor and delivery, eight times more likely to get caught in the birth canal, four times more likely to need resuscitation, four times more likely to become infected and thirty times more likely to be permanently injured.

A study conducted by Lewis E. Mehl, M.D., of the University of Wisconsin Infant Development Center reviewed 2,000 births. Nearly half of these had been home deliveries. Fourteen of the home-born babies had to be resuscitated as compared to fifty-two of those born in the hospital. And only one home-delivered baby suffered neurological damage compared to six of the hospital babies.

The figures reveal the benefits of home delivery. This is why many chiropractors and their families select natural childbirth at home.

In 1987, the German medical journal, *Manuelle Medizin*, published a report of a study which examined 1,250 babies five days after birth. Of this group, 211 suffered from vomiting, hyperactivity and sleeplessness. Upon examin-ation, 95 percent of these children had spinal abnormalities. After being adjusted, all the infants became quiet, the crying stopped, their muscles relaxed and they went to sleep.

The same report said that they found over 1,000 infants with nerve interference in the upper neck area which caused a variety of clinical conditions, ranging from central motor impairment to lowered resistance to infections, especially those of the ears, nose and throat.

In one case history, an eighteen-month-old boy suffered from tonsillitis, frequent enteritis, conjunctivitis, colds and earaches. Because of all these ailments he had trouble sleeping. After his first spinal adjustment, the little boy began to sleep through the night and it wasn't long before he was in good health.

Scientists are still learning how to accurately assess the damage to infants. They do know that a slight pull on the neck during delivery can cause a subluxation that might cause damage too slight to be noticeable immediately. But eventually it might cause some learning disability.

One of the greatest gifts you can give your newborn is a complete spinal examination by a doctor of chiropractic.

❈ ❈ ❈

CHIROPRACTIC FOR CHILDREN

Chiropractors feel strongly that the entire family can benefit by having spinal checkups.

The children who have been under regular chiropractic care get sick less often and less severely. They rarely miss days from school. Recent studies have also shown that they have fewer emotional and learning disabilities and other neurological problems connected with childhood.

In 1989, a study compared the patients of two-hundred pediatricians with two-hundred children who had been under the care of chiropractors. Not only was the overall health of the chiropractic children superior to those who had known only medical treatment, but they also had fewer ear infections, fewer allergies, lower incidence of tonsillitis and less need to be given antibiotic therapy.

❈ ❈ ❈

EAR INFECTIONS

Every parent has been awakened at some time during the night by the sound of a child crying from the agony of an ear infection. Usually, the culprit is a very painful condition called *acute otitis media*. The fever soars to 103 degrees or higher and fluid oozes out of the ear.

Most pediatricians will treat an ear infection with an antibiotic such as ampicillin or penicillin or an oral decongestant. Putting tubes in the ears and surgery on the eardrum (myringotomy) are used in severe cases. The problem is that every one of these treatments has negative side effects.

In the book *How to Raise a Healthy Child...In Spite of Your Doctor,* Dr. Robert S. Mendelsohn cites a double-blind study in which 171 children with acute otitis media were divided into four groups. The severity of the condition ranged from one ear to both ears being infected.

The first group received myringotomy surgery. The second group was given antibiotics. The third group was given a combination of surgery and antibiotics, and the fourth group received no chemical or surgical treatment at all. The authors of the study found that there was no significant difference between the four groups in terms of pain, temperature, discharge, otoscopic appearances or hearing loss. Furthermore, no one group suffered recurrences more than any other. In short, recovery was about the same for everyone, whether or not anything had been done.

Another study revealed that when antibiotics are given for ear infections, especially on the first day of the onset of infection, the disease isn't shortened by any measurable clinical standard. Antibiotics not only fail to cure the problem but they fail to prevent recurrence as well. In fact, recurrence rates were higher in children treated with antibiotic therapy.

Another common treatment for ear infections, mentioned on page 81, is a Tympanotomy which is a surgical procedure that inserts a tube in the ear of a child. This operation is so common it is performed over 1.2 million times each year. A British study examined patients who had received the tube in one ear but not in the other. Researchers showed that the eardrum with the tube tended to develop scar tissue that had the potential of leading to future hearing loss while the untreated ear healed normally without any problem. Although chiropractic doesn't treat ear infections. When a chiropractor corrects nerve interference, it often corrects a chemical imbalance, inviting the body to respond with its own powerful immune system. An eighteen-year study of 4,600 cases of upper respiratory infections in a core group of one-hundred families found that when spinal motion was restricted in the upper neck area, ear infection occurred. When spinal motion was maintained or re-established, complication usually didn't develop.

If your children have ear infections, chances are they have nerve interference, and you need to get them to a chiropractor for adjustments. When you do this, there is a good chance you will promote better health and also be able to avoid adverse drug reactions, side effects and allergic responses from medical treatments.

❄ ❄ ❄

TONSILS AND ADENOIDS

The tonsils are a very important part of the human immune system. They are two small lymph glands that sit at the back of the throat to protect us from infection and disease.

When the body fights infection, the tonsils can become enlarged and inflamed and covered with a white material. This condition, tonsillitis, is very painful. If tonsillitis is part of an upper respiratory infection, it's accompanied by a mild fever, cough, congestion and a runny nose. If it's the result of strep bacteria, there is a higher fever, the lymph glands in the neck become swollen and tender, and the breath may have a foul odor.

The adenoids are also lymph glands in the throat which fight disease. Unlike the tonsils, they are out of sight but they also serve to protect us from disease.

For several decades, tonsillectomies were one of the most common operations of childhood, with one-and-a-half to two-million being performed each year. In fact, there was a time when they were removed as just one of the "rites of passage." Unfortunately, the vast majority of the tonsillectomies were unnecessary. The only reason to ever remove adenoids or tonsils is because of a malignancy or airway obstruction caused by the tonsils swelling to the point where they have closed the throat and the child can't breathe. Any other reason for surgery is dangerous to your child's health.

Children's tonsils were most often removed to reduce the incidence of sore throats. However, sore throats involve a virus not bad tonsils. Removing the tonsils may pose more danger to the child's health. When the tonsils are gone, so is the child's first line of defense against infection. Now, the burden of fighting disease is transferred to the lymph nodes in the neck, which can lead to more dangerous complications.

Chiropractors know that it's perfectly normal for the body to host a certain amount of bacteria in the throat area without becoming ill. When your children are free from nerve interference, they will be better able to maintain a high level of natural immunity. A 1976 study showed that seventy of seventy-six children suffered from restricted movement in the upper neck area. Adjustments which resulted in correction of nerve interference allowed the children to fight off infection naturally and return to good health without complication.

❊ ❊ ❊

SCOLIOSIS

At some time during the early school years, almost every parent is asked to give permission for his or her child to have a scoliosis exam. Normally, everyone's spine curves slightly to the right or left and may even have vertebrae that manifest a little twisting or rotation. *Scoliosis* is an excessive curve or twist of the spine.

In most cases, the cause of scoliosis is unknown. Only ten-to-fifteen-percent of scoliosis cases can be traced to a tumor, infection, cerebral palsy, muscular dystrophy, disc problems or birth deformity.

Scoliosis isn't a terminal condition, and most people can lead a perfectly normal life without ever knowing they have it. In rare cases, where the scoliosis is more than thirty degrees, there may be impaired respiratory or heart function that's thought to be neurological in origin rather than mechanical.

The orthodox medical approach to scoliosis has undergone some changes. Before 1945, the body was encased in a plaster cast. Then doctors surgically used rods and metal restraints to straighten the spine. Other brace devices followed and then, electrical stimulation therapy became popular. Surgeons were quoted as saying that none of these methods did any good whatsoever. The newest research claims that ninety-five percent of all scoliosis patients can be identified by neurological tests, indicating the problem originates in the nerve system. Since chiropractors correct nerve interference, the best answer to the problem of scoliosis is to allow a chiropractor to adjust the vertebrae to correct the nerve interference which has caused or aggravated the condition.

❄ ❄ ❄

LEARNING DISORDERS

Current statistics indicate that eight million school children in the United States have a learning impairment, which can be traced back to some sort of malfunction in the nerve system.

When children have trouble learning, their frustration adversely affects their relationship with everyone around them—parents, siblings, teachers and schoolmates. Often, when a child develops a self-esteem problem, he or she is prone to emotional problems and psychological impairments that may carry into adulthood.

When children are hyperactive, due to emotional problems, medical treatment often includes medication, such as the drug, Ritalin, which has severe side effects. Ritalin doesn't always work and it often does more harm than good.

Recently, the director of Psychoeducational and Guidance Services of College Station, Texas, noted that out of 10,000 hyperactive children referred to him in the preceding decade, those who showed the most improvement had received chiropractic care. This caused the organization to refer some students to chiropractors for adjustments so they could monitor the effect of the care. Out of 24 students who had learning impairments, 12 received chiropractic care and the remaining students either received medication or no treatment at all.

The study concluded that chiropractic was twenty to forty percent more effective than the better known medications. Because students who are seriously afflicted seem to benefit so well from chiropractic, it seems inescapably logical that a "normal" child would benefit as well. It follows that chiropractic care can help an average student become above average. Perhaps a child's I.Q. can be raised—reading skills improved, etc. as well as being given an edge in alertness, coordination and speech.

"Chiropractors correct abnormalities of the intellect as well as those of the body."

D.D. Palmer

❄ ❄ ❄

CAN IT HELP MY CHILD?

"He knows when it flows above down, from inside out, naturally from the brain to the body, we are healthy and well."

B.J. Palmer, D.C.

We recommend all children be checked regularly for nerve interference, even without symptoms present. However, if you know a child who is not under chiropractic care and suffers from any of the following problems, please urge the child's parent's to consider chiropractic.

• Fever	• Headaches	• Neck Aches
• Colic	• Cough/colds	• Nervousness
• Croup	• Asthma	• Learning disorders
• Allergies	• Bed wetting	• Sinus problems
• Wheezing	• Bronchitis	• Eye problems
• Poor posture	• Constipation	• Scoliosis
• Stomach ache	• Weakness/fatigue	• Arthritis
• Hearing loss	• Ear infections	• Fatigue
• Neck/back pain	• Skin problems	• Pain in joints
• Leg/hip/foot pain	• One leg shorter	• Shoulder/arm pain
• Numbness	• Irritability	• Poor concentration

Parents who are aware of the importance of a properly functioning nerve system automatically want their children checked by a doctor of chiropractic.

Chapter 8

CHIROPRACTIC AND THE ELDERLY

Americans are living longer than ever before. In addition to living into our eighties and nineties, we're more active than we used to be.

The study of geriatrics, shows that it's possible to live a long, full life, and perhaps slow down the aging process.

Seniors can improve their strength, too. Dr. Maria Fiatarone affiliated with Tufts University and Harvard Medical School conducted a study in which nine seniors, ranging in age from eighty-six to ninety-six, worked out with a weight machine three times a week. They increased the strength of their quadriceps by an average of 174 percent. As one ninety-two-year old woman, said: "They made a new person out of me."

Not only is physical health maintainable, but so is mental health. In his best-selling book, *Quantum Healing*, Deepak Chopra states that:

"Careful study of healthy elderly people. . .has revealed that 80 percent of healthy Americans, barring psycho-

logical distress (such as loneliness, depression or lack of outside stimulation), suffer no significant memory loss as they age. The ability to retain new information can decline. . .but the ability to remember past events, called long-term memory, actually improves.

"As long as a person stays mentally active, he/she will remain as intelligent as in youth and middle age."

WHAT EXTENDS LIFE?

Gerontologists, scientists who study aging, now feel that life should continue to one-hundred or even one-hundred-twenty years, but they are surprised that so few make it. In 1995, the oldest woman in the world celebrated her 120th birthday and it was considered an unusual event around the world. While some centenarians are found to be drinkers and smokers, others shun tobacco and alcohol. Some are meat eaters and others are vegetarians. They can be religious or atheists. Many have led relatively easy lives, and there are some who have encountered tremendous difficulties. No one is quite certain what the magic ingredient is.

Studies have shown that the chances for longevity increase when people follow a low-fat, low-cholesterol, vegetarian diet and keep physically and mentally active. Furthermore, the subjects of these studies only visit a medical doctor on rare occasions.

THE MEDICAL APPROACH

Statistics show that there are 42.3 million people aged sixty and over living in the United States. Of these older adults, 9.6 million experience adverse reactions to prescribed and over-the-counter drugs every year. These reactions include drug-induced car accidents and falls, memory loss, parkinsonism, ulcers and death from overdoses of heart medicines and anesthetics. In 1991, people in this age group filled 650 million prescriptions—an average of slightly more than fifteen prescriptions per person.

In their book, *Worst Pills, Best Pills II* , Sidney M. Wolfe, M.D. and Rose-Ellen Hope, R.Ph., of the Public Citizen Health Research Group, expose the severe over-medication of our older citizens. Forty to fifty percent of the medications overused and mis-prescribed, especially tranquilizers (including sleeping pills and mind-altering drugs), cardiovascular drugs and gastrointestinal drugs. The medications that are used to treat heart disease, high blood pressure and vascular disease were found to be the most abused.

Older adults make up one-sixth (16.7%) of the population. This 16.7% of the population uses:

> **33.3% of all tranquilizers**
>
> **50% of all sleeping pills**
>
> **33.3% of all antidepressants**
>
> **65% of all high blood pressure drugs**
>
> **84% of all blood vessel dilating drugs**
>
> **43% of all gastro-intestinal drugs**
>
> **20% of all cold, cough, allergy and asthma drugs**
>
> **33% of all arthritis drugs**

Many older adults are happy to take medication to relieve their aches and pains. The medical community and the drug industry has also led them to believe these drugs will extend their lives.

Doctors often share the belief that an office visit should end by writing a prescription for an elderly patient. They may not know a great deal about geriatric medicine and they may fail to realize the danger drugs may have.on these adults. Too often, these older citizens go to more than one physician and get medication for different problems from each doctor. The combination of the various chemicals can be deadly.

Furthermore, when doctors who treated Medicare patients were tested about their knowledge of prescribing medicine for these patients, a study revealed that seventy percent of them did not pass. Ironically, the majority of the M.D.s who were asked to be in the study refused to take the test at all. They said they had no interest in the subject of geriatrics and medication!

The drug companies are often guilty of inadequate testing. Nevertheless, they market the drugs to M.D.s, sometimes using skewed test results, misleading claims and slick advertising. The Food and Drug Administration (FDA) conducted a study in which it found that of 425 drugs commonly taken by older patients, only 212 had proper geriatric dosage and contraindication information supplied with them.

The risk of a bad reaction to drugs is thirty-three percent higher in those between fifty and fifty-nine than it is in people in their forties or younger. The FDA has reported that most of the deaths from prescribed drugs occured in people who were sixty and over.

Here are some statistics from the World Health Organization regarding a study on adverse reactions to drugs.

88% of all people had at least one problem with a prescribed drug.

22% of these patients had a possibly life-threatening condition perhaps caused by medication.

59% were given drugs that were either ineffective or countra-indicated.

28% were given an incorrect high dosage.

48% were given drugs that had severe interaction effects when taken with other chemicals.

20% were given drugs that had the same effect of other drugs they were already taking.

According to a 1993 report entitled, *Arthritis, Rheumatic Diseases, and Related Disorders*, published by The National Institutes of Health, more than 37 million Americans are afflicted by one or more of the rheumatic diseases. In addition, more than 25 million Americans have osteoporosis, and countless millions have other musculoskeletal disorders. The fact to remember is that drugs are not the first answer to physical problems. Drugs should be used as a last resort when all other natural methods fail.

"Chiropractic is the only science that exactly locates the cause of the dis-ease, then adjusts it."

B. J. Palmer, D.C.

The drugs prescribed by medical doctors have serious side effects. For instance, aspirin may reduce pain and inflammation, but the sufferer may have to take eight or more tablets each day. This can cause stomach irritation, bleeding and ulcers. The non-steroidal anti-inflammatory drugs, such as Indocin, Advil and Naprosyn can cause kidney impairment, irritation and hemorrhage of the esophagus, stomach, duodenum and small intestine.

Doctors also prescribe steroids freely. Drugs like Prednisone and Hydrocortisone may offer some relief, but they make bones thin and weak. Gold Salts reduce inflammation, but they can create skin rashes and mouth ulcers.

"If you rush to take it (a new drug), do so with the full knowledge that you are being a guinea pig. The longer a drug is on the market, the more will be known about the side effects."

Robert S. Mendelsohn, M.D.

NOTE: In April 1982, Eli Lily introduced Oraflex. It was removed from the market in August 1982 after seventy-three people died from the effects of the drug.

Medicine doesn't have an answer to the very real problem of osteoporosis, high blood pressure, menopause and other conditions associated with aging. For instance, menopausal women in their forties and fifties, are given estrogen replacement therapy (ERT). By giving women small doses of the hormone estrogen, medical doctors have been able to slow bone loss but not renew bone mass.

Furthermore, ERT can create serious long term side effects, including an increased risk of breast cancer.

Another chemical therapy that's often prescribed to women is fluoride treatment. Not only is this non-effective; it also makes the bones more susceptible to fracture.

❄ ❄ ❄

THE CHIROPRACTIC APPROACH

The fact is the elderly need to be under the care of a chiropractor. When the chiropractor eliminates or reduces a patient's nerve interference, all the person's life support systems are strengthened and healing can occur naturally.

"There is no effect without a cause. Chiropractors adjust causes. Others treat effects."

B.J. Palmer, D.C.

When 250 million people believe in a bad idea, it's *STILL* a bad idea.

Chapter 9

A DEDICATION

To the Late Robert S. Mendelsohn, M.D.

Throughout this book, I have quoted from the works of a remarkable physician who was both an inspiration and a mentor to me. Robert S. Mendelsohn, M.D., was a physician but he became an outspoken detractor of the medical profession. In 1979, he published his best-selling book, *Confessions of a Medical Heretic*. He began it by saying: *I do not believe in modern medicine. I am a medical heretic. My aim in this book is to persuade you to become a heretic, too.*

Robert Mendelsohn raised a strong voice against the traditional hierarchy—and he knew what he was talking about. He was Director of Project Head Start's Medical Consultation Service and Chairman of the Medical Licensing Committee for the State of Illinois. He was honored numerous times with rewards for excellence in medicine and medical instruction. An advocate of a woman's right to have the best health care possible for herself and her child, he promoted home birth and spearheaded the grassroots' movement back to midwives who made house calls to help with the delivery. In addition to *Confessions of a Medical Heretic*, he also wrote *Mal-e*

Practice . . .How Doctors Manipulate Women, and *How to Raise a Healthy Child . . . in Spite of Your Doctor.*

He called hospitals *Temples of Doom* and advised people to stay out of them at all costs, especially when a new baby was involved. In *Mal-e Practice* he said:

An expectant mother should thank Providence for her good fortune if she has her baby in a taxicab on the way to the hospital. The cab driver may not be much help, but at least he will spare her from all of the purposeless, perilous, and unpleasant intervention her obstetrician had planned to inflict on her.

He said that after a lifetime of working in them, he found hospitals to be the "dirtiest and most deadly places in town." He pointed out that every year approximately 1.5 million people contract infections in the hospital, prolonging their stay—but they are luckier than the 15,000 who die of the infection. He said doctors downplay this, calling the condition a *nosocomial infection* rather than the more accurate *hospital-acquired infection.*

Throughout his distinguished career, Dr. Mendelsohn was always ready to play David to Modern Medicine's Goliath.

As controversial as he was in the 1970s and 1980s, today more and more of his theories are being validated. The movement towards fewer drugs, more natural healing and a naturally healthy lifestyle is a tribute to this man who was not afraid to speak out at a time when few were ready to listen.

Since the beginning of my career, I have considered Robert Mendelsohn to be a real hero to all of us who have promoted natural healing first before resorting to drugs or surgery.

It was sometime in the late 1970s, at a television talk show in St. Louis, Missouri, that I first met Dr. Mendelsohn. My wife and I were seated in the front row of the audience and Dr. Mendelsohn was a guest along with a local radiologist. They had both been asked on the program to debate the many issues Dr. Mendelsohn discussed in his books.

This was at a time too, when I was just beginning to speak out on radio and television shows across the country. I knew instantly that I could learn a lot from this distinguished doctor who dared to forthrightly criticize the institution of Modern Medicine, of which he was, at the same time, an esteemed—and yet, an openly despised—member. I admired Dr. Mendelsohn, too, because he spoke for Americans who were the victims of chemical and surgical "overkill."

After the show, I expressed my gratitude to him for what he was doing. I saw the strength and courage he had to have to confront the *status quo* in his profession when he believed they were wrong. Dr. Mendelsohn's memory still inspires me as I try to follow his example in my own profession, praising the good and exposing the bad. And at those times when I am being ridiculed for doing so, I remember Dr. Robert Mendelsohn and smile.

❈ ❈ ❈

Winifred Gardella's Experience

In the early 1950s Winifred Gardella was a poster child for the March of Dimes. Her picture was published in the newspapers to raise huge sums of money for the March of Dimes in San Francisco. Nationally, her image raised

99

millions of dollars to help fight the dreaded crippler, polio. Her sad, innocent face and her tiny body supported on crutches and leg braces, made many Americans reach into their pockets to donate.

But the March of Dimes couldn't help Winifred. After two and a half years under their doctor's expert care, her parents were told: "There is no hope."

Despite this dire prediction, her grandparents were determined to find a cure. They were not about to accept the opinion of so-called "medical experts." They decided to choose their own health care and they took Winifred to Dr. Lewis Robertson, a chiropractor. In less than six months of having her nerve interference corrected, Winifred Gardella threw away her crutches and braces and went for a walk with her chiropractor. She has been walking ever since!

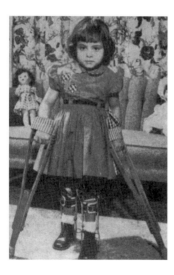

"March of Dimes" said there was no hope. Little Winifred would always have to use crutches and braces.

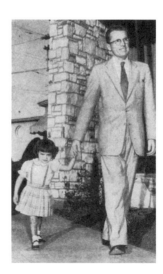

The once helpless little girl walks with her chiropractor.

Chapter 10

CHIROPRACTIC RESEARCH

The chiropractic profession has always relied on clinical research and experimentation. As we approach the 21st Century, chiropractic research is occurring around the world. Also, the chiropractic colleges are active in research as are several excellent research organizations which adhere to the strictest scientific standards. This chapter presents a sampling of some of the most noteworthy research studies conducted since 1980.

◆ At Michigan's Oakland University, Miron Stano, Ph.D., compared the health care costs for medical and chiropractic patients. By reviewing the insurance claims paid, Dr. Stano concluded that patients who received chiropractic care, either alone or in conjunction with medical care, experienced health care costs that were $1000 lower on average than those who received only medical care. Total insurance payments for patients who received only medical care were thirty percent higher than those who were under the care of a chiropractor. This lower cost was attributed to lower in-patient and out-patient costs and showed that "the chiropractic care substitutes for other forms of out-patient care."

◆ The Manga Report, from the University of Ottawa, reviewed all the international evidence on the management and low cost of back pain care. Pran Manga, Ph.D. concluded that significant cost savings would occur if the management of low back pain were transferred from physicians to chiropractors. He determined that chiropractic is safer than medical management of low back pain. "Many medical therapies are of questionable validity or are clearly inadequate. Chiropractic care is greatly superior to medical treatment in terms of scientific validity, safety, cost effectiveness and patient satisfaction." Dr. Manga concluded that "chiropractic should be fully insured (and) fully integrated into the Ontario health care system."

◆ The British Medical Research Council documented a ten-year study which compared chiropractic and hospital out-patient management of seventy-four patients with acute and chronic mechanical low back pain. The results showed that chiropractic care was significantly more effective than medical treatment for patients with chronic and severe pain. Furthermore, these results were long-term and remained consistent throughout the two year follow-up period. Chiropractic was also shown to save the British more than 10 million pounds a year by having hospital out-patients with low back pain under chiropractic care.

◆ These findings reinforced the conclusions of the New Zealand Report (377 pages) which was one of the most thorough and positive studies of chiropractic care on record. The twenty-month project was conducted by a government commission.

It concluded that spinal adjusting is a vital, very safe and clinically effective form of health care. Chiropractors have more thorough training in spinal mechanics and spinal care than any other health professional. Furthermore, chiropractic is scientifically based and must be made an integral part of all hospital care. Finally, the report said that "modern chiropractic is a soundly based and valuable branch of health care in a specialized area neglected by the medical professional."

◆ J.S. Wright, D.C., conducted a study and reported to the *Journal of Chiropractic* that 74.6 percent of patients with recurring headaches, including migraines, were either cured or experienced reduced headache symptoms after receiving chiropractic adjustments. Daniel C. Cherkin, Ph.D. and Frederick A. MacCormack, Ph.D., administered a survey in 1989 that concluded that patients who were receiving care from health maintenance organizations (HMOs) in Washington State were three times as likely to report satisfaction with chiropractic care as they were from other physicians. The patients also reported they believed that their chiropractor was concerned about their welfare.

1992 Statistic:	
Doctors in U.S.	Malpractice Premiums
Medical doctors	$41,971,000,000
Doctors of chiropractic	$62,500,000

◆ AV MED, a large HMO in the southeast, wanted to see if it could save money by having patients visit chiropractors for back pain. They chose one-hundred patients, eighty of whom had already been treated medically—without results. In each case, the patient had been seen by an average of 1.8 M.D.s. After receiving chiropractic adjustments, not one of the 100 patients had to have surgery. Furthermore, 86 percent of them got better and none of them got worse. Herbert Davis, M.D., the medical director of AV MED, said that chiropractic care saved the HMO $250,000 in surgical costs alone!

◆ The State Industrial Insurance Systems (SIIS) in Nevada compared the average medical and chiropractic care for patients who suffered industrial injuries from 1988-1990. The results showed that 24.4 percent were back injuries but they accounted for more than 50 percent of all medical costs. Over the three-year period, the average medical cost per patient was $2,142 which was 260 percent higher than the average chiropractic cost per patient of $892.

Loss of work time under chiropractic care is less than one-third that for medical care. Furthermore, injured workers are able to continue working while receiving chiropractic care which may not be an option for medical care patients who are advised to have bed rest and medication. The Nevada Worker's Compensation Study emphasized that chiropractic eliminates the concern and expense of inappropriate hospitalization, unnecessary surgery, improper use of medication including the high dosage of narcotic painkillers.

◆ In 1985, the University of Saskatchewan Study monitored 283 patients "who had not responded to previous conservative or operative treatment" and who were initially classified as totally disabled. The study revealed that after daily spinal adjustments were administered, "81 percent ...became symptom-free or achieved a state of mild intermittent pain with no work restrictions."

◆ The *British Medical Journal* reported in the June 2, 1990 issue that T.W. Meade, M.D. studied patients over a two-year period. Dr. Meade found that "for patients with low-back pain in whom spinal adjustments are not contraindicated, chiropractic almost certainly confers worthwhile, long-term benefit in comparison with hospital outpatient management."

◆ In 1991, Steve Wolk, Ph.D., studied 10,652 worker's compensation cases in Florida.The results reported by the Foundation for Chiropractic Education and Research concluded that: "A claimant with a back-related injury, when initially cared for by a chiropractor versus a medical doctor, is less likely to become temporarily disabled, or if disabled, remains disabled for a shorter period of time; and claimants treated by medical doctors were hospitalized at a much higher rate than claimants cared for by chiropractors."

◆ The Gallup Organization conducted a demographic

poll in 1991 which revealed that ninety percent of chiropractic patients felt their care was effective. More than eighty percent were satisfied with the care they received and almost seventy-five percent felt most of their expectations had been met during chiropractic visits.

◆ Also in 1991, Joanne Nyiendo, Ph.D., conducted a worker's compensation study in Oregon. She concluded that the median time loss in days for comparable injuries on any case was 9.0 days for patients who received chiropractic care as compared to 11.5 days for those who received medical treatment.

◆ Two years later, in 1993, researchers at the Royal University Hospital in Saskatchewan concluded that "the care of lumbar intervertebral disk herniation by side posture adjustments is both safe and effective." The researchers involved in the report, J. David Cassidy, D.C.; Haymo Thiel, D.C.; M.S. and W. Kirkaldy-Willis, M.D., are all on staff at the hospital's Back Pain Clinic.

◆ A 1992 review of data gathered from over two million users of chiropractic care in the United States appeared in the *Journal of American Health Policy*. It stated that "chiropractic users tend to have substantially lower total health care costs." The data also indicated that chiropractic care reduces the need for both physician and hospital care.

◆ *The Agency for Health Care Policy and Research (AHCPR) issues guidelines for low back problems.*

The U.S. agency for Health Care Policy and Research (AHCPR) formed a 23-person panel to find out the best ways to care for low back problems in adults. These health care professionals, including experts in orthopedic surgery, family practice, internal medicine, physical and rehabilitative medicine, emergency medicine, neurosurgery, rheumatology, and many other disciplines reviewed more than 3,900 studies on the topic. These guidelines released in December 1994 verified what chiropractors had been saying for years: surgery and medication should be a last resort treatment for most cases. Moderate exercise and chiropractic adjustments are far more effective and less risky.

Philip R. Lee, M.D. assistant secretary for health and director of the Public Health Service, said, "By encouraging people with acute low back problems to resume normal activities, using only those treatments that have been scientifically shown to be effective, these guidelines could save Americans considerable anguish, time and money now spent on unneeded or unproven medical care."

One clear message from all these studies is that chiropractic remains a cost effective and efficient method of healing that is, in many instances, equal or superior to medical care. The studies, which have often been conducted by state health or workers compensation agencies, have shown that chiropractic is often less expensive, significantly reduces the time away from work and often eliminates the dangers of drugs and surgery.

According to a 1991 report by the Harvard Medical Practice Study Group in Cambridge, Massachusetts: 80,000 persons die every year—one person every 7 minutes—and 150,000 to 300,000 more are injured annually from medical negligence in hospitals.

A Measure of Malpractice, **Harvard University Press 1993**

By now you know health doesn't come in a bottle. However, the pharmaceutical companies want you to believe that reaching for their lotions, potions, powders and syrups will make you healthy. All it does is make them wealthy.
Health comes from the inside out not the outside in.

Chapter 11

FREEDOM OF CHOICE

It's clear that when it comes to health care, the United States is anything but "the land of the free."

On every front, consumers and non-allopathic health care providers are struggling against a repressive and profit driven system which rivals George Orwell's worst "Big Brother" nightmare. Long ago the pharmaceutical and insurance industries formed an alliance with the medical establishment. Despite the court ordered truce that resulted from the Wilk case (see Chapter 12) these health care industries are continuing their push to discredit any methods or ideas which might loosen their stranglehold on the American public.

One report after another in the news media shows the medical/pharmaceutical/insurance monopoly targeting chiropractors. This establishment doesn't want doctors of chiropractic to threaten their complete control. Chiropractic currently represents only three-tenths of one percent of the total annual expenditure on health care in the U.S.

As if they didn't have enough power, the medical community has also enlisted the help of an equally formidable opponent: the United States government! On every level—local, state and even federal—our rights to make personal and family health care decisions have been usurped. This violates our fundamental rights to "Life, liberty and the pursuit of happiness." Millions of Americans are lied to every year regarding medications. Encouraged by our government officials, the message is enthusiastically broadcasted by the local and national media.

❄ ❄ ❄

NOT SMART ENOUGH?

If you should decide to choose treatment outside the organized and approved hierarchy of medicine, you will find it harder and harder to get insurance. You'll even get less compassion and understanding.

Stand at the border and watch the AIDS and cancer patients leaving for Mexico and Europe in hopes of finding treatment that doesn't exist in the States. We are denied access here to new medications and therapies, even when the condition has been diagnosed as terminal. Why? What's even more disturbing is medically aligned bureaucrats won't fully recognize chiropractic care, until we are shown to be scientifically validated. This sounds reasonable until you realize our government has hardly funded any research projects for chiropractic when compared to medicine.

Unfortunately, many medical treatment guidelines are devised by bureaucrats and claims adjusters and not by health care professionals. The over-riding consideration is financial instead of humanitarian. The pharmaceutical industry also adds to the problem. Physicians continue to prescribe drugs, because if they didn't the billion dollar pharmaceutical industry would not survive.

Many are aware of this situation. It's a very real concern and an accurate assessment of the situation in America. Many chiropractors also believe our profession is often attacked by medicine and the media to divert the public's attention away from the very real and well documented dangers of drugs and surgery.

※　※　※

THERE'S NO "PROOF IN THE PUDDING"

"Only 15% of all medical procedures are scientifically validated."

David Eddy, M.D., Ph.D.

Dr. David Eddy was the J. Alexander McMahon Professor of Health Policy and Management at Duke University in Raleigh-Durham, North Carolina. He received his M.D. degree from the University of Virginia and a Ph.D. in engineering economic systems at Stanford University in Palo Alto, California. After serving on the faculty at Stanford as a professor of engineering and medicine, he went to Duke University in 1981 to set up the Center for Health Policy Research and Education. Dr. Eddy has developed policies for a number of organizations, including the American Cancer Society, the National Cancer Institute, the World Health Organization, the Congressional Office of Technology Assessment, The Blue Cross and Blue Shield Association and the American Medical Association. His mathematical model of cancer screening was awarded the Lanchester Prize, the top award in the field of operations research. Dr. Eddy serves on the Board of Mathematics of the National Academy of Sciences and is a member of the Institute of Medicine.

When a man with Dr. Eddy's credentials claims that eighty-five percent of medical procedures have no scientific validation, it is important to the non-medical community to question the efficacy of modern medical practices.

❋ ❋ ❋

M.D.s ONLY

Examine the directors serving in the health care agencies at any level of government. Most likely, you'll see a hierarchy that's completely dominated by M.D.s.

The question is: Who's making the critical decisions about our future health care? Average citizens, including parents, doctors of chiropractic, or other alternative practitioners? No, the decision makers are Johnson & Johnson, Squibb, Merck, and all the other drug companies supported by the insurance companies who resist paying claims for anything outside the traditional medical venue.

SALES FIGURES FROM SECOND QUARTER, 1993

Company	Sales	Percentage increase over 1st Quarter sales
Johnson & Johnson	$3 billion	+ 9%
Squibb (domestic)	$2.7 billion	+12%
Eli Lilly	$1.4 billion	+12%
The Upjohn Co.	$859 million	+34%
Merck & Co.	$556 million	+12%
American Home Products	$265 million	+14%

These figures are for only three months April-May-June!

In the first half of the 20th century many chiropractors went to jail for practicing their art. In spite of past battles with organized medicine, our future is bright. Chiropractic is the largest non-medical healing system in the entire world. This incredible "American Discovery" is now flourishing as we approach the next century, but if we want natural health care to be available, we must be vigilant and protect our freedom of choice.

❄ ❄ ❄

Dr. Harry Llewellyn's Experience

I was reading when I first felt a dull ache in my lower back. The ache continued on and off for days. I knew that a car accident in my childhood had caused a severe lordosis or abnormal inward curvature of the lumbar vertebrae, but the injury had never affected me until now. Being a medical doctor, I followed the typical route of back x-rays and orthopedic surgeons. I was told I could avoid lying down on my back, tolerate the pain or try surgery. Not one of these answers appealed to me.

My brother-in-law advised me to visit a chiropractor. After a month of adjustments, I could read without any back pain. After five months of adjustments, I drove 18 hours back to New Jersey without any back pain. Until then, my limit in a car was 30 minutes.

It's not the rapid recovery from pain that amazes me. It's my profession. As a medical doctor, I had been an "alleged" non-believer in chiropractic. However, now I obviously believe in it. The pain in my right sacroiliac joint is gone. My knowledge of anatomy, physiology and biochemistry only strengthen my anticipation of the day when chiropractic is the brother of medicine.

Chapter 12

THE WILK v. AMA CASE

I t was a legal battle that continued for more than a decade. It was taken to the United States Supreme Court and finally, a multi-million dollar Federal Appeals Court decision was rendered against the American Medical Association (AMA) and forever changed the course of health care in this country.

Nevertheless, a lot of people have never heard of *Wilk et al vs. AMA*. Some might say this is because it lacked the drama of a Perry Mason courtroom or an episode of *L. A. Law*. Perhaps the antitrust issues were too complex for the general public to understand. There are some who claim the powerful medical establishment suppressed the news. No one will ever know for sure.

❄ ❄ ❄

THE VERDICT WAS "GUILTY!"

The guilty verdict in this case was as an indictment of the

AMA's lengthy attempt to illegally boycott the chiropractic profession.

The case began in 1976 when an Illinois chiropractor, Chester Wilk, and four other D.C.s filed a restraint of trade complaint against the American Medical Association. At that time, the AMA labeled all chiropractors as "quacks" and went so far as to forbid its members from associating with them.

Working with investigators, the five chiropractors found evidence that the AMA's stand was motivated by economics. Chiropractors, along with other forms of alternative health care were becoming strong competitors in the health care marketplace. The AMA wanted to stop these "invaders" who threatened their turf.

❄ ❄ ❄

A CAMPAIGN TO DESTROY

Throughout the years, as the case went through the courts, evidence mounted that the AMA had waged a systematic campaign to destroy the credibility of any alternative care health profession, particularly chiropractic. The worst part of this campaign was that people's health was affected—it was the patients who suffered the most.

On February 7, 1990, then US. Court of Appeals Judge, Susan Getzendanner, upheld a District Court's decision which found the AMA guilty of conspiring with other medical health care organizations in a "lengthy, systematic, successful and unlawful boycott" designed to restrict cooperation between M.D.'s and chiropractors in order to eliminate the profession of chiropractic as a competitor in the United States Health Care System.

The AMA appealed the case to the United States Supreme Court, but it was rejected. Judge Getzendanner's ruling stood.

The AMA complied with the court order and published the entire ruling in the *Journal of the American Medical Association* (JAMA) and the *American Medical News*. It also notified its members that they were free to refer to, accept referrals from, and associate with chiropractors.

❄ ❄ ❄

M.D.s & D.C.s WORK TOGETHER

Long before the AMA lifted its ban, medical doctors who weren't members of the Association had begun to establish good business relationships with their chiropractic colleagues.

Judge Getzendanner rejected the AMA's "medical patient care" defense and cited scientific studies which proved that "chiropractic care was twice as effective as medical care in relieving many painful conditions of the neck and back, as well as related musculo-skeletal problems."

Since the court's findings and conclusions were released, an increasing number of medical doctors, hospitals and health care organizations in the United States have begun to include the services of chiropractors.

While it's going to take time for some diehards in medicine to overcome their earlier negative indoctrination and personal prejudice about the "evils" of chiropractic—an alternative health care discipline—the Wilk case has opened the door for enhanced communication and cooperation between the two disciplines.

✻ ✻ ✻

"We never know how far-reaching something we may think, say, or do today will affect the lives of millions tomorrow."

B.J. Palmer, D.C.

Chapter 13

THE OTHER DRUG PROBLEM

Because of its concern with the health of all people, the World Chiropractic Alliance (WCA) has become very active in the war on street drugs. The WCA is involved in community activities aimed at increasing public awareness about the dangers of illegal drugs and engaged in a campaign to raise awareness of the legal drug problem worldwide. The legal drug problem is the misuse and abuse of prescription and over-the-counter (OTC) drugs.

While doctors of chiropractic recognize the value of some medications to relieve suffering or sustain life, doctors of chiropractic are almost unanimous in agreeing that, as a society, we take medications far too freely.

❈ ❈ ❈

WORSE THAN COCAINE!

Although it seldom receives media attention, the *other drug problem* (prescription and OTC drugs) takes a larger toll, in terms of lives, health and money, than all the illegal hard drugs combined.

The current edition of the *Complete Drug Reference* contains thousands of different medications. According to the FDA, there are hundreds of different OTC drug products available. Almost every one of these drugs, whether it's prescription or accessible over-the-counter, it can produce harmful side effects. Furthermore, many are highly addictive. One study showed that it's easier to get hooked on the commonly prescribed tranquilizer, Valium, than on cocaine or heroin.

❄ ❄ ❄

HOW SAFE IS SAFE?

The truth is that even so-called "safe" drugs aren't totally harmless. In an average twelve-month period, more than 1.5 million hospitalized people suffer from the side effects of the drugs and therapy they receive there. Aspirin alone sends about 1,600 people to the hospital each year who die from gastric bleeding.

Drug interaction also creates a serious problem. Some individual drugs may be relatively benign, but taken together, they can be deadly. According to the U.S. Department of Health and Human Services, the average American senior citizen is given more than fifteen prescriptions each year. Sometimes, these come from doctors who aren't aware of the other medications the patient may be taking. This could lead to tragedy if the drugs cause a toxic reaction.

All the drugs in the world cannot adjust a subluxated vertebrae.

B.J. Palmer, D.C.

❋ ❋ ❋

WHO'S TO BLAME?

Why is the legal drug situation out of hand? We know that in the United States the medical doctors are part of the problem because they write 1.6 billion drug prescriptions each year. In seventy-five percent of all office visits to an M.D. drugs are prescribed.

However, patients too, have to shoulder part of the blame. They seldom question their doctors and rarely request drug-free care, probably because most want a "quick fix" rather than a slower, more sensible approach to health.

Finally, a great deal of blame falls to the multi-billion dollar pharmaceutical industry which spends more than $10 billion each year to market its products which is much more than they spend on researching the safety of taking these drugs.

It's clear the legal drug problem is driving the cost of health care up and the level of health down. Use of drugs also sends a dangerous message to our youth. Every time we put a pill in our mouths to calm stress, stop headaches, wake up or go to sleep, etc., we are telling our young people that "it's okay."

NOTE: If the tranquilizer, Prozac, is a reasonable alternative to dealing with problems, how much of a reach is it to use marijuana or cocaine or worse?

121

Whether or not parents admit it, adults design the paradigms. It's the pattern we set that our kids follow. The next time you pop a pill, stop and consider what you're telling your children! It's up to you!

"Loss of life does not come from chiropractic adjustments: wish that we could say as much for surgical operations."

B.J. Palmer, D.C.

The most dangerous part of receiving chiropractic care, is driving your motor vehicle in traffic to the chiropractic office.

Chapter 14

WHO USES CHIROPRACTIC?

As stated before, Chiropractic is for everyone, not just blue collar workers injured on the job, athletes with pulled muscles, accident survivors with whiplash, the very young or the elderly. Every year, more and more people of all ages and from all walks of life are turning to chiropractors to improve their performance. Ballerinas and quarterbacks. . . movie stars and politicians. . . golfers and singers . . heavy weight champs and royalty are all among chiropractic's celebrity patients, past and present.

❊ ❊ ❊

CHIROPRACTIC PATIENTS

BASEBALL: Ryne Sandberg, Brett Butler, Wes Parker, Don Sutton, Jeff Reardon, Roberto Clemente, Rick Monday.

BASKETBALL: Robert Parish, Jack Sikma.

BEACH VOLLEYBALL: Craig Moothart, Sinjin Smith,

Kent Steffes, Tim Hovland, Randy Stoklos.

BODYBUILDERS: Arnold Schwarzenegger, Lori Ugolik, Franco Columbo, D.C.

BOXERS: Evander Holyfield, Jack Dempsey, Rocky Marciano, Tony Lopez, Michael Carbajol.

DANCERS: Marcello Angelini, Daniella Buson.

ENDURANCE ATHLETES: Biathletes—Kenny Sousa, Joel Thompson, Brent Steiner and Fred Klevan. **Triathletes**—Mark Allen, Craig Reynolds and Larry Rhoads.

ENTERTAINERS: Arnold Schwarzenegger, Shirley Mac-Laine, Mel Gibson, Meredith Baxter, Liza Minnelli, Bob Hope, Doris Day, Glen Campbell, the band Alabama, Rosanne Cash, Dixie Carter, Madonna, Cher, Linda Hamilton, Dennis Weaver, Richard Gere, Kim Bassinger, Alec Baldwin, Whoopie Goldberg, Ted Danson, Macaulay Culkin, Burt Reynolds.

FOOTBALL: Dammone Johnson, Alex Karras, Ricky Bell, Joe Montana, Mark Mays.

GOLFERS: Barbara Bunkowsky, Jan Stephenson, Amy Alcott, Donna White, Kim Bauer.

HOLLYWOOD STUNTMAN: Russell Towery.

OLYMPIC ATHLETES: Joseph Arvay (wrestling), Mary Lou Retton (gymnastics), Bruce Jenner (decathlon), Alberto Juantorena (400 & 800 meter run), Dwight Stones (high jump), Suzy Chaffee (skiing).

ROYALTY: Princess Diana of England.

RUGBY: Terrence Titus

SKEET: Louise Kolar Terry

SOCCER: Brian Haynes, Gregg Blasingame.

SURFER: Jeff Booth.

TENNIS: Tracy Austin, Jimmy Connors, Billie Jean King, John McEnroe, Ivan Lendl.

There are at least 25 million other people who are enjoying the benefits of regular chiropractic health care. If you are not one of them you need to ask yourself, why not? You cannot believe that you are doing everything for you and your family's health if chiropractic care is not included in your life or your family's.

Please don't take your health for granted. Unfortunately, it is difficult for any individual to fully appreciate his or her health until it's gone, and when this happens the first symptom may be the last one i.e. heart attack, stroke or kidney failure. Remember symptoms are the last thing to appear in a disease process.

Please, if you or your family have not been screened for nerve interference make an appointment today and make the effort to improve your health!

Chapter 15

THE CHIROPRACTIC PRINCIPLES

Chiropractic has many basic principles upon which all its philosophy, art and science is based. Those listed here are some of the most important. They have guided the profession since its earliest development. Some of them are almost universally accepted. Others are just beginning to find acceptance with other sciences. These principles follow a simple progression of deductive logic. If you accept the major premise, the other principles fall into place almost automatically.

❄ ❄ ❄

THE MAJOR PREMISE

A Universal Intelligence is in all matter and continually gives to it all its properties and actions, thus maintaining it in existence.

❄ ❄ ❄

THE SECONDARY PRINCIPLES

◆ The expression of this Intelligence through matter is the chiropractic meaning of life.

◆ Life is a Triune having three necessary united factors, namely, Intelligence, Force and Matter.

◆ In order to have 100% Life, there must be 100% Intelligence, 100% Force, 100% Matter.

◆ A living thing has an Inborn Intelligence within its body, called Innate Intelligence.

◆ The mission of Innate Intelligence is to maintain the material of the body in active organization.

◆ There is 100% of Innate Intelligence in every living thing, the required amount, proportional to its organization. The amount of force created by Intelligence is always 100%.

◆ The function of Innate Intelligence is to adapt universal forces and matter for use in the body, so that all parts of the body will have coordinated action for mutual benefit.

◆ Innate Intelligence adapts forces and matter for the body, but is limited by the limitations of matter.

The forces of Innate Intelligence will never injure or destroy the structures in which they work.

◆ The forces of Innate Intelligence operate through or over the nervous system in animal bodies.

◆ There can be interference with the transmission of Innate Forces.

◆ Interference with the transmission of Innate Forces causes dis-ease.

❄ ❄ ❄

I AM A CHIROPRACTOR

I am a Chiropractor working with the sciences of the universe by turning on the life in man thru the art of the adjustment. I do not prescribe, treat or diagnose conditions. I use only my hands. I work with that "mysterious something" which created my body from two cells.

At a time prescribed aeons ago I was set in this body to experience. That cosmic power which created me, which also moves the seas, rotates the earth, directs the heavens, gives life, takes it away, is everything. And that power which set the universe in motion and created me did not abandon me when I became free of the security of my earthly mother's womb. It is still with me and protects me as it moves all forms toward their final predestined goal.

It is not mine to educatedly ask "why" or "where", but to Innately live; and live to help my fellow creatures. And with this Chiropractic adjustment I use all the powers and energies moving this universe, to allow my fellow creatures the chance to live, free of dis-ease.

I wish nothing in return, only the chance to GIVE. I give with the only thing I have, LOVE. And I love all by removing that which interferes with 100% of LIFE. I do not look to others for direction, I look within. I am a perfect expression of God living 24 hours each day for others — I am a PRINCIPLED CHIROPRACTOR.

B. J. Palmer, D.C., Ph.C.

❄ ❄ ❄

129

THE BIG IDEA

A slip on the snowy sidewalk in winter is a small thing. It happens to millions.

A fall from a ladder in the summer is a small thing. It also happens to millions.

The slip or fall produces a subluxation. The subluxation is a small thing.

The subluxation produces pressure on a nerve. That pressure is a small thing.

That decreased flowing produces a dis-eased body and brain. That is a big thing to that man.

Multiply that sick man by a thousand, and you control the physical and mental welfare of a city.

Multiply that man by one hundred thirty million, and you forecast and can prophesy the physical and mental status of a nation.

So the slip or fall, the subluxation, pressure, flow of mental images and dis-ease are big enough to control the thoughts and actions of a nation.

Now comes a man. And one man is a small thing.

This man gives an adjustment. The adjustment is a small thing.

The adjustment replaces the subluxation. That is a small thing.

The adjusted subluxation releases pressure upon nerves. That is a small thing.

The released pressure restores health to a man. This is a big thing to that man.

Multiply that well man by a thousand, and you step up the physical and mental welfare of a city.

Multiply that well man by a million, and you increase the efficiency of a state.

Multiply that well man by a hundred thirty million, and you have produced a healthy, wealthy, and better race for posterity.

So, the adjustment of the subluxation to release pressure upon nerves, to restore mental impulse flow, to restore health, is big enough to rebuild the thoughts and actions of the world.

The idea that knows the cause, that can correct the cause of dis-ease, is one of the biggest ideas known. Without it, nations fall; with it, nations rise.

This idea is the biggest I know of.

B. J. Palmer, 1944

B. J.'S LAST PRINTED WORDS

Time always has and always will perpetuate those methods which better serve mankind. Chiropractic is no exception to that rule. My illustrious father placed this trust in my keeping, to keep it pure and unsullied or defamed. I pass it on to you unstained, to protect as he would have you do. As he passed on, so will I. We admonish you to keep this principle and practice unadulterated and unmixed. Humanity needed then what he gave us. You need now what I give you. Out there in those great open spaces are multitudes seeking what you possess.

The burdens are heavy; responsibilities are many; obligations are providential; but the satisfaction of traveling the populated highways and byways, relieving suffering and adding millions of years to lives of millions of suffering people, will bring forth satisfaction and glories with greater blessings than you think. Time is of the essence.

May God flow from above-down His bounteous strengths, courage and understanding to carry on; and may your Innates receive and act on that free flow of Wisdom from above-down; inside-out...for you have in your possession a Sacred Trust. Guard it well.

GLOSSARY

ADJUSTMENT: The specific application of forces used to facilitate the body's correction of nerve interference.

ALLOPATHIC: Refers to conventional medicine as practiced by the graduate of a medical school which grants a medical degree.

ALVEOLI: Air cells of the lungs.

ANTIBODIES: Proteins manufactured by lymphocytes to neutralize foreign protein, such as bacteria, viruses and other microorganisms in the body.

BASAL GANGLIA: Four masses of gray matter located deep within the brain.

CAPILLARIES: Small blood vessels.

CATATONIC: An unresponsive person refusing to move or talk, remaining in a fixed posture.

CEREBELLUM: A large portion of the brain connected to the brain stem and spinal cord. It coordinates voluntary muscular movements.

CEREBRUM: The largest portion of the brain consisting of two hemispheres. It receives information from the senses—sight, hearing, taste, and smell—through the brain stem and processes the data. It also deals with the higher mental faculties, such as thinking and comprehension.

CHIROPRACTIC: A primary health care profession in which professional responsibility and authority are focused on the anatomy of the spine and immediate articulation, and the condition of nerve interference. It is also a practice which encompasses educating, advising about and addressing nerve interference.

CHIROPRACTIC CARE LEVELS: There are three levels of care you will progress through when you are under the care of a doctor of chiropractic. The length of each care level is at the discretion of the practitioner and varies from patient to patient.

> **Level I Care:** A patient-specific number of visits, from daily to three times a week, with the objective of beginning the reduction of the clinical indicators of nerve interference. The duration of Level I care is at the discretion of the practitioner.

> **Level II Care:** A patient-specific number of visits, from one to two times a week beginning with the first reduction of the clinical indicators of nerve interference with the objective of reducing clinical indicators to a minimum level. The duration of Level II care is at the discretion of the practitioner.

> **Level III Care:** This is lifetime care with the frequency of office visits varying depending on the patient. It begins with the maximum reduction of the clinical indicators of nerve interference, and has the objective of sustaining the patient at that level.

CHIROPRACTIC DIAGNOSIS: A comprehensive process of evaluation of the spinal column and its immediate articulations to determine the presence of nerve interference and other conditions that may contraindicate chiropractic procedures. (See Medical Diagnosis .)

CHIROPRACTIC PRACTICE OBJECTIVE: The professional practice objective of chiropractic is to correct nerve interference in a safe, effective manner. The correction is not considered to be a specific cure for any particular symptom or disease. It is applicable to any patient who exhibits nerve interference regardless of the presence or absence of symptoms or disease.

DEDUCTIVE LOGIC: The Chiropractic Principle is based on this process of reasoning. A process of reasoning in which the conclusion follows necessarily from the major premise presented.

DIS-EASE: The word *disease* is a combination of *dis* and *ease*. *Dis* is a prefix meaning "apart from." It follows then that dis-ease is nothing more than a lack of comfort, a loss of harmony in the system. Chiropractors believe that instead of treating disease with chemicals and invasive procedures, whenever possible, first treat dis-ease with the reduction or elimination of nerve interference, thereby giving the patient a chance to recover naturally before resorting to drugs and surgery.

COMPENSATORY: To make up for or counterbalance.

EOSINOPHIL: A type of cell of the peripheral blood or bone marrow whose granules stain red with eosin or other acid dyes.

EPIDERMIS: The outermost layer of skin.

ESTROGEN: Female sex hormones, estradiol and estrone, produced by the ovary. Responsible for the development of secondary sexual characteristics.

FIBRIN: A protein necessary for cells to form clots.

HEALTH: A state of optimal physical, mental and social well-being; not merely the absence of disease or infirmity.

HOMEOPATHY: A system of medicine, founded by Dr. Hahnemann in 1796 in Philadelphia, in which drugs are used in extremely small doses.

HOMEOSTASIS: The ability or tendency to maintain normal, internal stability and balance in an organism by coordinated responses of the organ systems. Examples of homeostatic mechanisms are the regulation of blood pressure, body temperature and blood sugar levels.

HYDROCHLORIC ACID: Normal constituent of gastric juice found in the stomach. Produced by the parietal cells of the gastric glands to serve many digestive functions.

HYPERACTIVE: Beyond or above normal behavior, excessive movements.

HYPERKINETIC: Excessive amounts of mobility. Similar to hypermobile.

LARYNX: The enlarged upper end of the trachea known as the organ of voice. It consists of nine cartilages bound together by an elastic membrane moved by surrounding muscles.

LEUKOCYTE: A cell that acts as a scavenger and by so doing helps combat infection.

LETHARGY: A condition of sluggishness.

LIGAMENT: A band or sheet of connective tissue between the ends of bones that facilitate motion and support.

LYMPH NODES: A rounded body of lymphatic tissue of varying sizes, that produce lymphocytes and monocytes. They act as filters to keep bacteria from entering the blood stream. They also may stop cancer cells, but in turn may be the seat of cancer.

MANIPULATION: The forceful passive movement of a joint beyond its active limit of motion. It doesn't imply the use of precision, specificity or the correction of nerve interference. Therefore, it is not synonymous with chiropractic adjustment.

MARROW: Tissue inside the long bones of the body. Red marrow is involved with the production of blood cells.

MAST CELLS: Cells which are present in most body tissues but most prevalent in connective tissue, such as the innermost layer of the skin. They play an important role in the body's allergic response because they release chemicals responsible for allergic symptoms into the tissue.

MEDICAL DIAGNOSIS: Procedures that provide information about disease processes for the selection of treatment.

MEDULLA OBLONGATA: The lower portion of the brain stem and the enlarged part of the spinal cord in the skull.

MELANIN: The pigment which gives color to hair and skin, etc.

METABOLISM: The rate and sum of all the physical and chemical changes that take place within the body.

MRI: *Magnetic Resonance Imaging* or MRI uses a combination of radio waves, magnetic fields, and computers to create a high quality picture of the internal organs, the soft tissue and the nerve network. Like the CAT Scan, the patient lies motionless while being passed through a narrow cylinder. It can detect brain and spinal tumors, disc disease, spinal stenosis, degeneration and indications of a stroke. It's also used to examine heart and liver tissue and the joints. This is the method that is preferred for examination of spinal disc degeneration.

MYELOGRAPHY: The Myelogram procedure includes a "spinal tap" which is used to get information on spinal cord compression and disc problems. A needle is inserted between the lumbar vertebrae, spinal fluid is drained and replaced with dye, then the patient is X-rayed. There are risks inherent in this procedure Some patients may develop severe headaches that can last for several weeks or months. Others are allergic to the dye which can stay in the body for years. Furthermore, the results are not entirely accurate. Myelography is being replaced by MRI and CAT Scans.

NERVE INTERFERENCE: See vertebral subluxation.

NEUTROPHILS: A leukocyte which can be readily stained by neutral dyes.

NOSOCOMIAL INFECTION: An infection contracted as a result of being hospitalized.

OSTEOPATHY: Originally, a system of medicine based upon the theory that the normal body is able to rectify itself against toxic conditions. While some manipulation is still used to treat patients, most osteopaths today rely heavily on drugs and surgery to treat patients.

OSTEOPOROSIS: Increased porous condition of bones with bones becoming soft.

PAPILLAE: A small, nipplelike protuberance or elevation.

PARKINSONS: A chronic nerve disease characterized by a fine, slowly spreading tremor; muscular weakness and rigidity.

PARASPINAL EMG SCANNING: A painless, non-invasive procedure to measure and record the electrical signals given off by the muscles that attach to the spinal column. Electrodes are placed on the skin and their readings are shown in the form of a graph. Since one of the symptoms of nerve interference is abnormal muscle activity, the EMG is becoming a popular method for charting muscle spasms and spinal imbalance.

PEPSIN: The chief enzyme of gastric juice which converts proteins.

PHALANGES: The bones of a finger or toe.

PYLORUS: The lower opening of the stomach into the small intestines.

RENNIN: A Coagulating enzyme found in the stomach of cud-chewing animals which curdles milk.

TARSAL BONES: The seven bones of the ankle.

THERMOGRAPHY: This procedure measures the temperature on the skin surface to locate inflammation of muscles and soft tissues. A special camera takes pictures which reflect the different temperatures by displaying a range of colors on film. Thermography has been used to pinpoint spinal nerve and muscle stress.

TRIUNE OF LIFE: The name for the three elements which influence every living organism: Innate Intelligence, Innate Energy and Innate Matter.

VERTEBRAL SUBLUXATION: Also referred to as nerve interference, is a misalignment of one or more of the 24 vertebrae in the spinal column, which causes alteration of nerve function and interference to the transmission of mental impulses, resulting in a lessening of the body's Innate ability to express its maximum health potential.

VESTIGIAL: A bodily part or organ that is small and

degenerate or imperfectly developed in an earlier stage of the individual.

VITALISM: The doctrine that teaches that in living organisms, life is caused and sustained by a vital principle distinct from all physical and chemical forces. It also teaches that life is, at least in part, self-determining and self-evolving.

X-RAY: The common name for *Radiograph* which is a picture of the solid parts of the body produced by passing electromagnetic rays through the body positioned against photographic film. The rays pass through the soft tissues but are stopped by metal and other solid objects, like the bones including teeth. The X-ray tube was invented by Wilhelm Roentgen in 1895, the same year D. D. Palmer discovered chiropractic. His son, B.J. Palmer, established one of the finest X-ray laboratories in the country because he realized the contribution X-ray diagnosis would make to spinal analysis.

REFERENCES AND FOOTNOTES

I've intentionally not listed references or footnotes throughout the text. I wanted to avoid interfering with the concentration of the reader. Anyone interested enough to research the contents of this book will find the list of references to be more than adequate source material. These references are offered for suggested reading material as well as confirming the validity of the statements and contents of this book.

HISTORY OF CHIROPRACTIC

Dye, A. August: *The Evolution of Chiropractic: Its Discovery and Development*. Richmond Hall, Richmond Hill, NY 1969.

Maynard, Joseph E: *Healing Hands: The Official Biography of the Palmer Family*. Fourth Edition. Jonorm Publishers, Woodstock, GA 1991.

Moore, J. Stuart: *Chiropractic in America: The History of a Medical Alternative*. John Hopkins University Press, Baltimore, MD 1993.

CHIROPRACTIC PHILOSOPHY

Bach, Marcus: *The Chiropractic Story.* DeVorss & Co. Los Angeles, CA 1968 reprinted by Si-Nel, Marietta, GA.

Barge, Fred H.: *Life Without Fear.* Barge Chiropractic Clinic, LaCrosse, WI.

Dintenfass, Julius: *Chiropractic: A Modern Way to Health.* Pyramid Books, NY 1975.

Koren, Tedd: *Bringing Out the Best in You.* Koren Publications, Philadelphia, PA 1994.

Koren, Tedd: *World's Greatest Drugstore.* Koren Publications, Philadelphia, PA 1977 and 1994.

Rutherford, Leonard W.: *The Role of Chiropractic.* Clinton Press, Inc., Erie, PA 1989.

Strauss, Joseph: *Your Amazing Body.* Lifeline Publications, Levitown, PA

HEALTH AND HEALING

Chopra, Deepak: *Quantum Healing.* Bantam Books, New York, NY 1989.

Moyers, Bill: *Healing and the Mind.* Doubleday, New York, NY 1993.

Siegle, Bernie: *Love, Medicine and Miracles.*

INSIGHTS ON TRADITIONAL MEDICINE

Carter, James P.: *Racketeering in Medicine.* Hampton Roads Publishing Company, Norfolk, VA 1993.

Inlander, Charles B., Leven, Lowell S., Weiner Ed: *Medicine on Trial.* Pantheon Books, New York, NY 1988.

Mendelsohn, Robert S.: *Confessions of a Medical Heretic.* Contemporary Books, Chicago, IL 1979.

Mendelsohn, Robert S.: *Malepractice.* Contemporary Books, Chicago, IL 1982.

Mendelsohn, Robert S.: *How to Raise a Healthy Child in Spite of Your Doctor.* Ballantine Books, New York, NY 1984.

Schmidt, Michael A., Smith, Lendon H., Sehnert, Keith W.: *Beyond Antibiotics.* North Atlantic Books, Berkeley, CA 1993.

Speransky, A.D.: *A Basis for the Theory of Medicine.* Translated and edited by C.P. Dutt. New York International Publishers 334, 1943.

Szasz, Thomas: *The Theology of Medicine.* Syracruse University Press, Syracruse, NY 1988.

Wolfe, Sidney M.: *Worst Pills Best Pills.* Public Citizen Health Research Group, Washington, DC 1988.

CHILDREN AND CHIROPRACTIC

Biedermann H.: Kinematic Imbalances Due To Suboccipital Strain In Newborns. *Manual Medicine* 6(5):151, 1992.

Briegel, Louis R., Stefanski, Stacey A.: *For the Love of Children.* Innate Publishing, Canton, GA 1993.

Blessing S.J.: What You Should Know About Ritalin. *Chiropractic Pediatrics* 1(1):16, April 1994.

Collins K. F., Barker C, Brantley J. et al: The Efficacy Of Upper Cervical Chiropractic Care On Children And Adults With Cerebral Palsy: A Preliminary Report. *Chiropractic Pediatrics* 1(1):13, April 1994.

Golden L., Van Egmond C.: Longitudinal Clinical Case Study: Multi-disciplinary Care Of Child With Multiple

Functional And Developmental Disorders. *J Manipulative Physiol Ther* 17(4):279, 1994.

Goodman, R., Mosby J.: Cessation Of A Seizure Disorder: Correction Of The Atlas Subluxation Complex. *Journal of Chiropractic Research and Clinical Investigation* 6(2):26, Feb 1991.

Gutmann G.: Blocked Atlantal Nerve Syndrome In Infants And Small Children. English translation in *International Review of Chiropractic* 46(4):37, July 19990. Original German paper published in *Manuelle Medizin* 25:5, 1987.

Klougart N., Nilsson N., Jacobsen J.: Infantile Colic Treated By Chiropractors: a prospective study of 316 cases. *J Manipulative Physiol Ther* 12:281, 1989.

Koren Tedd: Muscular Dystrophy and Chiropractic: The Eric Knapp Story. *Chiropractic Pediatrics* 1(1):18, April 1994.

Langley C.: Epileptic Seizures, Nocturnal Enuresis, ADD. *Chiropractic Pediatrics* 1(1):22, April 1994.

Marko R.: *Bed Wetting: Two Case Studies. Chiropractic Pediatrics* 1(1):21, April 1994.

Masarsky C., Weber M.: Somatic Dyspnea And The Orthopedics Of Respiration. *Chiropractic Technique* 3(1):26, Feb 1991.

Phillips N.: Vertebral subluxation And Otitis Media: a case study. *Journal of Chiropractic Research and Clinical Investigation* 8(2):38, July 1992.

Rubinstein H.: Case Study: Autism. *Chiropractic Pediatrics* 1(1):23, April 1994.

Schimp J., Schimp D.: The Neuropathophysiology Of Traumatic Hemiparesis and Its Association With Dysfunctional Upper Cervical Motion Units: a case report. *Chiropractic Technique* 4(3):104, Aug 1992.

Schutte B., Teese H., Jamison J.: Chiropractic adjustments And Esophoria: a retrospective study and theoretical discussion. *J Manipulative Physiol Ther* 12:281, 1989.

Van Breda W., Van Breda J.: A Comparative Study Of The Health Status Of Children Raised Under The Health Care. *Journal of Chiropractic Research* 101, Summer 1989.

Woo C.: Post-traumatic Myelopathy Following Flopping High Jump: a pilot case of spinal manipulation. *J Manipulative Physiol Ther* 16(5):336, 1993.

IATROGENIC (DOCTOR CAUSED) ILLNESS

Bedell, S.E., Deitz, D.C., Leeman, D., Delbanco, T.L.: Incidence and Characteristics of Preventable Iatrogenic Cardiac Arrests. *JAMA* 265(21):2815, June 5, 1991.

Begley, Sharon: The End Of Antibiotics. *Newsweek*, March 28, 1994.

Dye, Michael: Silent Danger Of Medical Malpractice: third leading cause of preventable death in U.S. *Public Citizen* May/June 1994. Public Citizen Health Research Group, Washington, DC.

Evans, R.S., Classen, D.C., Stevens, L.E., Pestotnik, S.L., et. al.: Using a hospital information system to assess the effects adverse drug events. *Proc Annu Symp Comput Appl Med Care*: 161, 193.

Ferner, R.E., Whittington R.M.: Coroner's cases of death due to errors in prescribing or giving medicines or to adverse drug reactions: Birmingham 1986-1991. *J.R. Soc Med* 87(3):145, Mar 1994.

Stremple, J.F., Bross, D.S., Davis, C.L., McDonald G.O.: Comparison of Postoperative Mortality and Morbidity in VA and Nonfederal Hospitals. *J Surg Res* 56(5):405, May 1994.

Quires Torres, G., Hernandez, J., Reyes, A.: Iatrogenic Diseases in Surgery of the Ear. *Rev Laryngol Otol Rhinol (Bord)* 114(1):25, 1993.

Robin, E., McCauley, R.: The Malpractice Crisis and the Rate of Actual Malpractice. *Adm Radiol* 13(1):20, Jan 1994.

Stambouly, J.J., Pollack, M.M.: Iatrogenic Illness in Pediatric Critical Care. *Crit Care Med* 18(11):1248, Nov 1990.

Steel K., Gertman P.M., Crescenzi C., Anderson, J.: Iatrogenic illness on a general medical service at a university hospital. *New England Journal of Medicine* 304(11):638, Mar 12, 1981.

WORLD CHIROPRACTIC ALLIANCE

Is chiropractic and its drug-free approach to health care an important issue for you? Have you found relief, avoided surgery or discovered how your family can benefit from regular visits to your chiropractor to maintain wellness and build natural immunity?

Do you feel the government or insurance companies have the right to choose the type of health care you should have access to?

Even though chiropractic is the world's largest natural healing profession, unfair managed care programs, legislators and insurance companies are quickly closing the door on your freedom of choice regarding health care. This is clearly an organized effort to once again eliminate chiropractic as a health care choice for consumers.

The World Chiropractic Alliance (WCA) is a non-profit organization made up of chiropractors and chiropractic consumers. The purpose of the WCA is Promoting a Vertebral Subluxation Free World.

The WCA is a watchdog organization ready to challenge any group or organization that threatens the chiropractic practice objective. The WCA will fight any discrimination against chiropractic consumers. We need your help to protect your constitutional rights—your fundamental right to choose your mode of healthcare.

Index

- THE OFFICIAL -

Spanglish Dictionary

Un User's Guía to More Than 300 Words and Phrases That Aren't Exactly Español or Inglés

BILL CRUZ, BILL TECK, AND THE EDITORS OF
GENERATION Ñ MAGAZINE

ILLUSTRATIONS BY DAVID LE BATARD

A Fireside Book
Published by Simon & Schuster

Para our *familias*

FIRESIDE
Rockefeller Center
1230 Avenue of the Americas
New York, NY 10020

FIRESIDE and colophon are registered trademarks
of Simon & Schuster Inc.

Manufactured in the United States of America

10 9 8 7 6 5 4 3 2

Library of Congress Cataloging-in-Publication Data
Cruz, Bill.
    The official Spanglish dictionary : un user's guía to more
    than 200 words and phrases that aren't exactly español
    or inglés / Bill Cruz, Bill Teck and the editors of Generation Ñ ;
    illustrations by David Le Batard.
        p.   cm.
      1. Spanish language—Foreign elements—English—
    Glossaries, vocabularies, etc.   2. English language—
    Influence on Spanish—Glossaries, vocabularies, etc.
    3. Languages in contact—United States.   4. Cuban
    Americans—Language—Glossaries, vocabularies, etc.
    5. Cuban Americans—Language—Humor.   6. Languages
    in contact—United States—Humor.   I. Teck, Bill.
    II. Generación Ñ.   III. Title.
PC4827.C78   1998
462'.421—dc21   98-33688   CIP

ISBN 0-684-85412-0

ACKNOWLEDGMENTS

Special thanks to Josie Goitisolo, one particular angel without whom this book could not have existed. *Muchas Gracias.*

Thanks to our editor Becky Cabaza for her patience in waiting for returned *beepazos* (beeper calls) and *timrazos* (phone rings) and her understanding in regard to this whole process.

To Gustavo Perez-Firmat and Luis Santerio for inspiration.

To Dave Le Batard for the *sabroso* (yummy), gorgeous drawings that grace our book.

To Footy, Liz Balmaseda, and Lydia Martin for spreading Spanglish along the banks of the Swanni River.

To Raul Mateu: World's most dangerous agent.

The *Generation ñ* rogues' gallery (or how these writers and editors helped us win the war on proper language): Contributing to this book were: Annette Alvarez, Juan de la Luz, Ana Escribano, Maria Budet, and Lynn Norman. With a Special Sunday Night session by Benny Milán and Adriana Gonzalez. *Y gracias a* Delio Nunez Menocal for allowing us to bounce on *el trampolín de la confianza* and Ignacio Medrano for directions to Guashinton D.C. And Val Prieto for the following piece of Spanglish:

Saludiños (saludos con cariño).

BILL AND BILL

CONTENTS

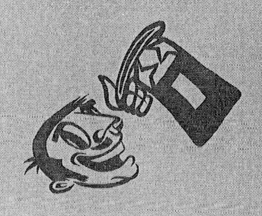

SAT ACROSS FROM MY MAN

READING *El Diario*

RIDING THE TRAIN DOWNTOWN

FROM *el barrio*

—The Beastie Boys, "B-Boy Bouillabaisse"

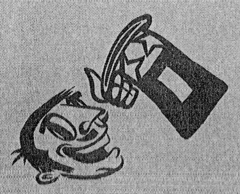

INTRODUCTION

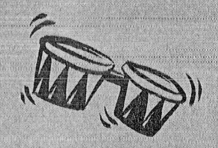

Spanglish is a strange thing. Like art (and some other stuff), you may not be able to describe it, but you know it when you see it. True Spanglish emerges when one switches from Spanish to English (or vice versa) within the same sentence. For example: "*No creo que voy* on the trip with you," which translates into, "I don't think I'm going on the trip with you."

Many Hispanics raised in this country, educated in American schools from grade school through college, primarily spoke Spanish with their families at home. As a result, Spanglish sentences like the one above are nothing short of commonplace. Everyday. Rudimentary. Nothing special. But, when we see one in print, it makes us laugh. It's the humor of recognition. And that's what brings us to this book. As the editors of *Generation ñ* magazine, and as Miami dwellers, we come into contact with Spanglish every day, in every setting, from the personal to the professional. In keeping an accessible, relaxed voice within our magazine, we allow ourselves the luxury of switching languages within our articles—sometimes there just isn't a word in English that *really* captures what we're trying to convey. In our attempts to meld both languages and capture the vibe of one culture in the tongue of another (whether it be on the pages of our magazine or at the corner drugstore), Spanglish emerges. And yet, it is still bigger than this. . . . We're going to attempt to come up with a more deep-seated meaning for Spanglish.

Spanglish dates back to the time when Spanish and Anglo-Saxon societies first came into contact with one another, and especially in the New World, where rumor has it that descendants of Cabeza de Vaca insisted their name meant "head of state," and not "head of cow." It has permeated pop culture from the song "Que Será, Será" and Ricky Ricardo's riffs on his wacky wife ("LuCY! You got song esplaining to do!"), down to the many e-mail exchanges written in Spanish where folks tell each other that they will look *en la Web* (on the Web) for a document or upload it from *el harddrive* (you get the picture), when what they mean is *la red del internet* or *el disco duro*.

The use of Spanglish is quite pervasive in popular music. Everyone from Xavier Cugat and Carmen Miranda to Sam the Sham and the Pharaohs with "Woolly Bully" (with the great Spanglish count off: "one, two, one, two, *tres, cuatro* . . .") and Gloria Estefan with "Mama Yo No Go" (a song about a daughter coming to terms with the difference between her and her mother's relationship to their homeland), has creatively toyed with the differences between

Spanish and English, expressing certain concepts in either language (or a mixture of the two) because they sound richer, or merely for effect. Spanglish has never, however, been written about or seriously cataloged in a way that zeroes in on how humorous some of these words really are.

To simply pitch a switch up in languages is something a lot of us do in daily life, which brings us to the strange categorizations in our little book. Some of these words are straight translations; some are transliterations, both textual and verbal as well as modified; some are descriptive; and some are just the traditional adoptions of language that we Latinos have been doing merrily for years. It's not enough for the word to be mispronounced or articulated with an accent—its meaning has to bend or alter in some way or the mispronunciation has to replace the word in daily usage even among people who know it's not correct.

Miami is the town that inspired the bilingual sitcom *¿Qué Pasa USA?* It's the town where Gloria Estefan recorded "Conga," her English-language Latin conga song. It's the place where Raúl Alfonso of the legendary charanga group Hansel y Raúl screamed at the end of their first album's extended closing jam, "*¡Se acabó el disco, y lo acabamos en budget!*"—meaning, "the record is over, and we finished it within budget!" There isn't a word in Spanish that captures the rigid feel of the word "budget." That's where true Spanglish comes from: When a word from English is more descriptive than a phrase in the mother tongue and replaces it. For example, Latinos never say "salary," and not just to avoid confusion with "celery." They say *suerdo*, meaning what a person earns, the correct word in the right place. No sweat. But when the manager comes around he remains just that, in English or Spanish. We'd never refer to a *gerente director* but we would tell *el manayer* that we were calling in sick.

So this book was born in Miami's *cafeterías* and little ol' American hardware stores, where *abuelos* of both cultures just try to get along. This is what we got. You see, to be Cuban is to be in a hurry much of the time, we think. And to live in exile is to be a little off-center sometimes. Our story is that we rushed through life, flying on shots of caffeine, with nothing to lose and everything to gain. We made up Miami as we went along. And we communicated the best we could with the time we had. Kind of half-assed, I guess.

What time did we have for correct elocution? We'd started mangling and realigning English words back in Cuba, and that was one custom exile wasn't gonna take from us. This was always something I'd taken for granted, until Bill Cruz showed me (and all of us) how extraordinary it was.

To realize what's special about your culture and validate it—through song, word, painting, or cataloging—is really something. Gustavo Perez-Firmat, Willy Chirino, Alvarez Guedes, the Shull Sisters, and the folks at the Cuban American Library at the University of Miami are just some of the champions of *lo nuestro*. To be able to see what's around you and dissect it in an interesting and funny way is a gift few people have. Cruz has it.

When we met at Versailles (Miami's formost *cafetería*) for *un cafecito*, I had just started *Generation ñ*, a magazine geared toward Cuban Americans, and as I sat there and listened as he explained his ideas, I thought, "Well, I hope people like this." He had a collection of words that were unique to our culture and he was pretty sure people would get it, but he seemed eager and confident, and not being one to look a gift horse in the mouth, I said, "What the heck."

The response, of course was—and is—overwhelming. Everywhere I go, people tell me that their favorite part of the magazine is "the page where you list the words." We never thought that the most popular aspect of our publication would be one we never planned, but it certainly is. *La gente* love it and they constantly let us know—writing, faxing, e-mailing, and calling with suggestions and kudos.

After pitching our idea to turn his column into a humor book for Simon & Schuster's Fireside imprint, we agreed that the thing to do was to make this tome a little less Cuban and a little more Latino in flavor, resulting in the most Cuban thing we've done. We tried to expand it, tried to make it an all-encompassing look at Hispanic Spanglish, but you know what? We're two insular kids from Miami, this is who we are. And humor needs to be specific to be funny, so basically we went with the old axiom, "write what you know." And we did. It was the only way for us to be funny. This does, however, leave the door open to our Mexican-American, Puerto Rican, Dominican-American friends to come up with their own volumes of colloquial Spanglish. Latin culture is so diverse in this country in Spanish alone, but it's pretty different in Spanglish too. The recent Dominican independent film *Nueba Yol*, the awesome merengue raps of the Nuyorican band Proyecto Uno, the chart-busting rhythms and incredible lyrics of Tejeno music, the magazine *Latina*, John Leguizamo, and so much more all make Spanglish something that just ain't going away. And those are just some of the flavors out there.

Although these words are pretty funny, what also struck me as I was reading over our book was how touching these were, in a very peculiar way. Each generation holds on to yesterday's traditions while in some fashion coming to terms with a new society. This is us.

BILL TECK

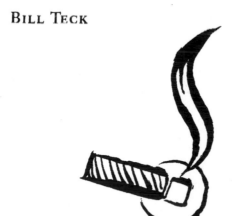

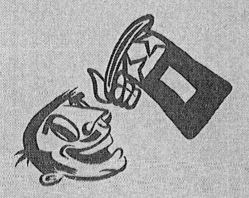

SAYINGS

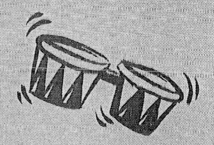

Before we get into the entries it's interesting to note the comical everyday translations that take place when Hispanics (*especially* Miamians) turn Spanish phrases into nonsensical English sayings that only they understand (and even then, just barely). Here's a sampling of just how descriptive and flowery the Spanish language can be, with each saying followed by the Spanish translation, then the actual meaning in English.

"He threw himself to the low income quarters."
Se tiró para el solar.
He got a little wild.

"His cables are crossed."
Él tiene los cables cruzados.
He's confused.

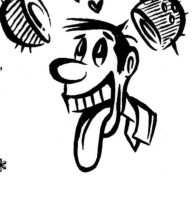

"He's got a coconut."
Él tiene un coco.
He's got a crush.

"He threw the house out the window!"
¡Botó la casa por la ventana!
That rocks!

"He's a postcard."
Es una postalita.
He's a pretty boy.

"Not even a goat can jump it."
Eso no lo brinca un chivo.
It's a big problem.

"He sandpapers himself."
Se da lisa.
He takes good care of himself.

"He sang the peanut vendor."
Cantó el manicero.
He died.

"She's very much a monkey."
Qué mona.
She's cute.

"He's a piece of bread."
Es un pan.
He's a good guy.

"He plays the dead fly."
"Se hace la mosquita muerta."
He plays dumb.

"He's the leg of the devil."
Es la pata del diablo.
He's trouble.

"Between, between and drink a chair."
Entre, entre y tome una silla.
Come in, come in and have a seat.

"For if the flies."
Por si las moscas.
Just in case.

"My hand left me."
Se me fue la mano.
I overdid it.

"I'm gonna enter you to clean crackers."
Te voy a entrar a limpiar galletas.
I'm going to slap you.

"He's running the ball."
Está corriendo la bola.
He's spreading a rumor.

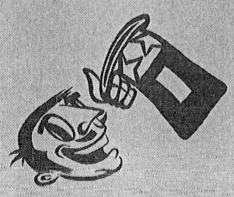

SPANGLISH
CLASSIFICATIONS

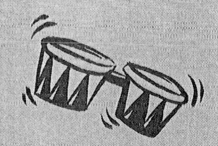

You'll notice that each Spanglish entry features a "class," which we've defined as one of the following:

TRANSLITERATION: By far the most popular of the classes, the transliteration is a phonetic adoption from another language. It's a "literal translation" of the way a word sounds to the listener. Transliterations are always born in the same way: a person (probably your *abuelo*) hears a foreign word for which there is no equivalent in his or her native tongue. The word or phrase is then mimicked as closely as possible, and, upon repeated use, is eventually incorporated into the language. In short, the transliteration is what makes it possible for the stock boy at Home Depot to understand that sheet rock is what Cheo needs when he asks, *"Oye, mijo, ¿dónde está el chirro?"*

DESCRIPTIVE: This is the simplest category used. Words classified as descriptive attempt to explain some aspect of the object or idea they identify. The reference is usually visual, but sometimes it can be taken further. Try asking for *un raspadito* next time you're at the window of a Cuban *cafetería*. It's easier than keeping track of whatever they're calling the scratch-off lotto tickets this week.

TRADITIONAL: These are the words that need no introduction. As far as we know, they've been around since the dawn of time. In other words, traditionals are *más viejos que andar a pie.* Enough said.

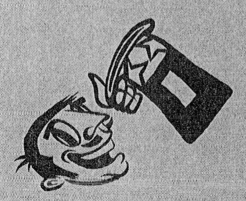

ON THE STREET

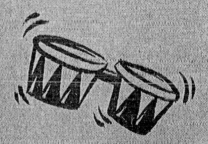

Places to go, people to see, neighborhoods to get lost in. Here's what happens when *Miamiengse* Latins take to the road.

el autopar n. the local auto parts shop, sacred temple of amateur Hispanic mechanics

    Class: Transliteration.

    Origin: I would dare say that this kidnapping of the term "auto parts" has been around for a long, long time. Remember, we are talking about Hispanics and car repair here.

    Typical usage: "Mire, señor, yo no vengo más a este autopar. ¿Qué le importa a usted si le cambio el aceite a mi carro en este parqueo?"

English: "Look, sir, I'm not coming back to this *autopar.* What the hell do you care if I do an oil change in your parking lot?"

Bosguagon *n.* the Volkswagen Beetle

Class: Transliteration.

Origin: This bit of Spanglish came about in the '60s as this economical automobile became the vehicle of choice for Hispanic hippies.

Typical usage: Cheo, if you don't shift this *Bosguagon* a little faster, we're gonna miss Santana at Woodstock.

marque *n.* a supermarket

Class: Transliteration.

Origin: Partial phonetic adoption of the English term.

Typical usage: "Vete pa'l marque y búscame unos encuentros de pollo."

English: "Go to the *marque* and get me some chicken legs and thighs."

gróceri *n.* grocery store or supermarket

Class: Transliteration.

Origin: Straight phonetic adoption.

Typical usage: "*Me vendieron un mamoncillo podrido en este gróceri. No me gasto ni un quilo prieto más aquí.*"

English: "They sold me a rotten mammonsillus in this *gróceri.* I won't spend another filthy cent here."

Guendis *n.* Wendy's fast-food restaurant

Class: Transliteration.

Origin: Forget that, you should hear Dave Thomas' Spanish.

Typical usage: "*Por qué le dirán Guendis a ese gordito de la corbata.*"

English: "I wonder why they call that fat guy with the tie *Guendis.*"

Berguerguín *n.* Burger King

Class: Modified transliteration.

Origin: This popular fast-food chain attracted

Latin customers with its reasonable prices and good food, especially the *Guáper* (Whopper), resulting in this tasty bit of Spanglish.

Typical usage: "It takes two hands to handle a guaper at *Berguerguín*."

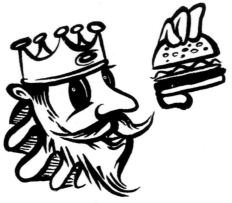

Macdónal *n.* McDonald's

Class: Transliteration.

Origin: Although most American refer to the fast-food mascot with the familiar Ronald, Hipanics simply refer to him as *Macdónal*, as if it were a first name.

Typical usage: "*Oye*, take a picture with *Macdónal*."

Pisa Ho n. Pizza Hut

Class: Transliteration.

Origin: The struggle to find a good family pizza place led Hispanics to this parlor of pepperoni.

Typical usage: "Come here, hon, and settle a bet between your mother and me. Is it *Pisa Hau,* or *Pisa Ho?*"

Sebenileben n. 7-Eleven convenience store

Class: Transliteration.

Origin: Needing a place to buy milk, Big Gulp, and Lotto tickets, the 7-Eleven stores became *Sebenileben.*

Typical usage: "*Oye, los hotdos de Sebenileben son muy ricos.*"

English: "Hey, the *hotdos* at *Sebenileben* taste yummy."

Berguerguín de Pollo n. Kentucky Fried Chicken

Class: Descriptive.

Origin: As certain uninformed Miami *abuelas*

assumed *Berguerguín* meant fast-food establishments, the attempt here was to signify that
this fast-food establishment served chicken.
Typical usage: "I'm not in the mood for a *jambergue,* just stop at *el Berguerguín de Pollo.*

El Pollo del Viejito n. Kentucky Fried Chicken
Class: Descriptive.
Origin: The man on the bucket (literally,
"The Little Old Man's Chicken").
Typical usage: "*Este pedazo de Pollo del
Viejito está un poco pasado de grasa. A mí me
gusta el crispi.*"
English: "This piece of *Pollo del Viejito* is a
little heavy on the grease. I like the Extra
Crispy."

**Don Jon Silva n. Long John Silver's fast-food
restaurant**
Class: Transliteration.
Origin: But they *look* like *croquetas.*
Typical usage: "*Qué bien hacía el papel de*

Sonny Croqueta en Miami Vice *el Don Jon Silva ese, pero qué raras son las croquetas de pescado en su restaurante."*

English: "That *Don Jon Silva* did a great job on *Miami Vice* as Sonny Crocket, but how weird are the fish croquettes at his restaurant."

guarejaus *n.* a warehouse

Class: Transliteration.

Origin: Furniture Warehouse, a Cuban-owned and operated furniture store in Miami whose radio spots coined the mispronunciation.

Typical usage: "El taller de Pepín está al lado de Furniture Guarejaus."

English: "Pepín's shop is right next to the Furniture *Guarejaus*."

pisicorre *n.* a station wagon

Class: Descriptive.

Origin: An oral contraction of the Spanish words *pisa y corre*, meaning "step and go." Since station wagons were among the first automobiles in Cuba to arrive with automatic transmissions installed (the feature that allows you to step and go), they were christened with this distinctive moniker.

Typical usage: "Chico, desde que fuimos a la playa la semana pasada no he podido sacarle la arena al pisicorre."

English: "Buddy, ever since we went to the beach last week, I haven't been able to get the sand out of the *pisicorre*."

paragüero *n.* **inept motorist**

Class: Traditional.

Origin: This word has its root in the word *paraguas* (umbrella). *Paragüero* was created when the correlation was made between older people's affinity for taking walks with umbrellas and the general perception of their driving skills.

Typical usage: "¡Paragüero!"

English: "Practice makes perfect."

sagüecera *n.* **Miami's southwest residential areas**

Class: Modified transliteration.

Origin: A term coined by Hialeah residents as their verbal revenge on all the "outsiders." Taken from the English word "southwest" and modified.

Typical usage: "*Dime tú, ¿que pinta fulano por la sagüecera?*"

English: "You tell me—what business does so-and-so have hanging around the *sagüecera?*"

jandi *n.* **a parking space reserved for the handicapped**

Class: Modified transliteration.

Origin: A $500 fine and a misunderstanding.

Typical usage: "*Voy a entrar y salir nada más, cuélate en el jandi dos minuticos.*"

English: "I'll be in and out—just sneak into the *jandi* for two minutes."

tique *n.* **ticket**

Class: Transliteration.

Origin: The parking meter attendant near your office.

Typical usage: "I can't believe *que me sonaron un tique* with time on the meter." (I got stuck with a ticket!)

Tensén *n.* **a reference to the now-defunct Woolworth's chain, or other similar retail establishments**

Class: Transliteration.

Origin: Taken from the English phrases "five-and-dime" and "five-and-ten-cent store."

Typical usage: "*Oye, vieja, voy un minutico al Tensén, que se acabó el Bibaporrú.*"

English: "Hey, honey, I'm going to the *Tensén* for a minute: we're out of Vick's Vapor Rub."

tranporteichon *n.* **barely adequate automobile**

Class: Transliteration.

Origin: Our parents lifted this one from the

term "public transportation." They realized—like everyone else does—that public transportation sucks, but it eventually gets you where you're going. It seemed only natural to use part of the term to describe a car that does the same thing.

Typical usage: "*Bueno, la verdad es que yo quería comprarme un Buique. Pero, imagínate tú, este carrito lo que me costó fueron 400 miserables pesos y—qué carajo—está bastante feito pero es un tranporteichon.*"

English: "Well, the truth is, I really wanted to get a Buick. But this car only cost me four-hundred miserable dollars. I mean, what the hell, I know it's ugly but it's a *tranporteichon*."

La Vaquita *n*. the closest Farm Stores to your house

Class: Descriptive.

Origin: A reference to the cow, or *vaquita*, found on the establishment's outdoor lighted sign.

Typical usage: "*Niña, anoche asaltaron al viejito que trabaja en La Vaquita.*"

English: "Last night they assaulted the little old guy that works at *La Vaquita*."

yipe *n.* rugged, four-wheel vehicle

Class: Transliteration.

Origin: A direct phonetic adoption except for the Spanish-like ending "e" sound. Please note that this word applies to the classic jeep-style vehicle, i.e., crashbar- or rag-top. Any newer Jeep model such as a Wrangler or Cherokee should be referred to as a *camioncito*.

Typical usage: "*Te crees tú que te vas a comprar un yipe, muchacho. Si te vuelcas en una de esas mierditas, te quedas en la página dos.*"

English: "Yeah, right, you think you're buying a Jeep, kid. If you overturn that little piece of crap, you'll stay on page two."

dauntaun *n.* urban downtown areas

Class: Transliteration.

Origin: As straight and simple as it gets, kids.

Typical usage: "*Cuando yo llegué al exilio, caminaba por el dauntaun de noche encantado de la vida. Pero ahora hay que estar loco de remate para andar por ese barrio. ¡No, hombre, no!*"

English: "When I first got to this city, I used to walk around *dauntaun* at night without a care in the world. Now you'd have to be insane to stroll through that neighborhood."

llompear *v.* the act of connecting two vehicles' power sources together with jumper cables in order to induce recharging of one of the vehicle's batteries

Class: Modified transliteration.

Origin: Taken from "jump" (as the process is commonly referred to in its abbreviated English form) and mock-conjugated into Spanish.

Typical usage: "*Oye, jefe, hazme el favor, ¿tienes cables? Que voy a llompear este cacharro de mierda por la última vez antes que lo tiro en un canal.*"

English: "Hey, chief, do me a favor, will you? Have you got cables? I need to *llompear* this crappy car one last time before I drive it into a canal."

parquear *v.* **the act of parking an automobile**

Class: Modified transliteration.

Origin: The English word "park" is used as a root and conjugated into almost every Spanish form imaginable: *parqueando, parqueaste, parquearon, parqueándose,* and so on.

Typical usage: "Mira a ver donde se te ocurre parquear el carro por el dauntaun, que si te descuidas te dejan con un alambre pelado y el timón."

English: "Careful where you decide to *parquear* your car around downtown. They'll leave you with a stripped wire and a steering wheel."

un sú *n.* **a legal suit**

Class: Modified transliteration.

Origin: Latinos have adapted to the American way of life as well as any other ethnic group, providing legal fodder for everything from the Supreme Court to Judge Wapner.

Typical usage: "Mira, mano, tú le diste a mi moto con el picop tuyo, pero yo tengo fulcober y te voy a meter un sú."

English: "Listen, buddy, you hit my *moto* (motorcycle) with your *picop* (pickup truck) but I have *fulcober* (full coverage) and am going to hit you with a suit."

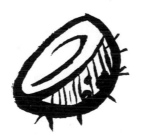

Lost in Translation No. 1

Try to match your favorite American cartoon character to their Hispanic alter ego

1) Popeye

2) Olive Oyl

3) Swee'pea

4) Wimpy

5) The Flintstones

6) The Jetsons

7) Donald Duck

8) Bugs Bunny

9) Elmer Fudd

10) Daffy Duck

11) Heckle and Jeckle, the talking magpies

12) Goofy

13) Quick Draw McGraw

a. *Elmer Gruñon*

b. *Popeye*

c. *Checho y Chucho, las uracas parlanchinas*

d. *Tribulín*

e. *Pilón*

f. *Los Supersónicos*

g. *El Pato Pascual*

h. *Coco Liso*

i. *El Conejo de la Suerte*

j. *Rosario*

k. *El Pato Loco*

l. *Tiro Loco McGraw*

m. *Los Picapiedra*

ANSWERS: 1) b; 2) j; 3) h; 4) e; 5) m; 6) f; 7) g; 8) i; 9) a; 10) k; 11) c; 12) d; 13) l

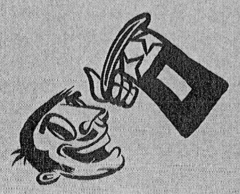

SEXUAL HEALING

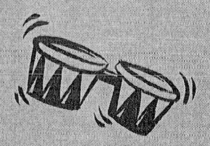

A little Barry White (or Nelson Ned) and, as Chef on *South Park* says, you've gotta set the mood. Ladies and gentleman, the international language:

fuiqui fuiqui n. sexual intercourse; copulation
> *Class:* Descriptive.
> *Origin:* A verbal mimicking of the sound and rhythm of an overworked, squeaky bed spring.
> *Typical usage: "Sube el televisor, Manolo, que los vecinos están haciendo fuiqui fuiqui otra vez."*
> *English:* "Turn up the TV, Manny, the neighbors are doing the *fuiqui fuiqui* again."

beibi *n.* amatory pet name; generic amorous sobriquet

> *Class:* Transliteration.
>
> *Origin:* Obviously, this one is directly transliterated from the English word "baby" (a term so firmly cemented in the romantic idiom of American pop culture that it is next to impossible to pinpoint exactly where or when it was appropriated by Hispanic-Americans).
>
> *Typical usage:* "*Ay, beibi, tú con tantas curvas y yo sin frenos.*"
>
> *English:* "Oh baby, you've got so many curves and I just lost my brakes."

sexi *adj.* sexy; sexually appealing

> *Class:* Transliteration.
>
> *Origin:* Phonetic adoption of the English word "sexy."
>
> *Typical usage:* "*Ese escote está muy sexi para una vieja con tanto jamón.*"
>
> *English:* "That plunging neckline is a little too sexy for a lady with that much ham on her."

Piropos/Come-Ons

Si cocinas como caminas, me como hasta la raspita.

If you cook as good as you look, I'll scrape the bottom of the bowl.

Te llevo de rama en rama, como Tarzán lleva a Juana.

I'll swing you from branch to branch, like Tarzan takes Jane.

Estás como Santa Bárbara: santa por delante y bárbara por detrás!

You're like Saint Barbara (*bárbara* = amazing)— saintly up front, amazing from behind.

A ti no te duelen ni los callos.

You're so fine even your bunions don't hurt.

¡Arroz! ¡Carne hay!

Bring the rice! We've got the meat!

Hombre:	*¿Te dolió?*
Mujer:	*¿Qué me dolió?*
Hombre:	*Cuando te caíste del cielo, mi ángel.*
Guy:	Did it hurt?
Girl:	Did what hurt?
Guy:	When you fell from heaven, my angel.

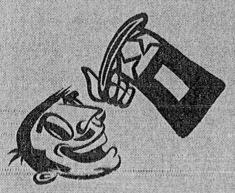

INSULTS AND
TERMS OF
ENDEARMENT

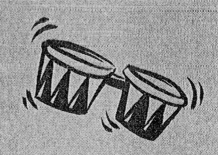

"Idiot." "Imbecile." These words easily translate to *idiota* and *imbecil*. But there are other terms, somewhat more Spanglish-esque, that we use to address our loved (and not-so-loved) ones. They are as follows.

broder n. **brother**

    Class: Modified transliteration.

    Origin: Power to the people, or something like that.

    Typical usage: "¡Oye, broder!"

    English: "Hey, bro!"

chipero n. **one who is reluctant or unwilling to utilize personal finances**

Class: Modified transliteration.

Origin: Rooted in the English word "cheap," "*chipero*" evolved out of the need for a more street-level term for a tightwad, or *tacaño*. The Spanish suffix "*ero*" or "*era*" is commonly used to affiliate an occupation or lifestyle to an individual, i.e., a *manicero* is a peanut vendor; a *callejera* is a woman who is always out on the streets; and a *chipero* is *un tipo que camina con los codos*.

Typical usage: "Don't be such a *chipero*, man, we're tired of eating taco supremes!"

friquiado adj. **in a state of nervousness or shock; behaving erratically**

Class: Modified transliteration.

Origin: Taken from the English phrase "Ahhhh, FREAK OUT!" Actually, it's an adaptation of "freaked out" that came about at the height of the freak-based-phrase era. (Yeah, you remember.) We just couldn't resist dragging this one into our Spanglish conversations to replace less colorful terms.

Typical usage: "El perrito mío está friquiado desde que le hicieron la operación. Cada vez que enciendo el televisor, se mea."

English: "My doggie is *friquiado* ever since he had the surgery. Every time I turn on the TV, he starts to pee."

fula (1) *n.* a foolish person (2) *n.* an American dollar bill in Cuba

Class: (1) Transliteration; (2) Traditional.

Origin: (1) Hispanics looking for a good substitute for idiot, modified the word fool for Spanish usage. (2) The word "moolah" combined with Fidelism means a reliance on the *fula*, a disdainful word for the American dollar, as well as an expression of disdain for the U.S. presence in Cuba.

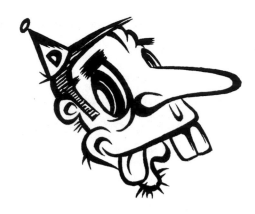

Typical usage: (1) "Bro, you really are a tremendous *fula*." (2) *Mira, asere, préstame un fula para el taxi.*

English: (2) "Hey buddy, lend me a dollar for the cab."

Mandraque *n.* **magician possessing supernatural powers; a mystic**

Class: Transliteration.

Origin: The source of this word can be traced to "Mandrake the Magician," a King Features comic that first appeared in 1934. Aside from his telepathic powers and mysterious demeanor, the main appeal for Hispanics was that his physical features made him look like one of us. Of course, he wasn't really Hispanic, it was just an illusion.

Typical usage: "*Mijita, el horóscopo de ayer decía que iba a tener éxito en el trabajo y hoy me aumentaron el sueldo. No es por nada, pero la verdad que ese Walter es un Mandraque cualquiera.*"

English: "Let me tell you, yesterday's horoscope said I was going to succeed at work, and I just got a raise. Honestly, girl, that Walter* is a modern-day *Mandraque*."

saramambich adj. son of a bitch

Class: Transliteration.

Origin: *Tío* Cuco's first U.S. driving experience.

Typical usage: Watch where you going, you *saramambich!*

---

*A reference to Walter Mercado, the flamboyant undisputed king of Latino astrology. (Think Shirley MacLaine meets Dionne Warwick meets Liberace, and you'll get the idea.)

Insults

Si ese se cae, coma yerba: If he falls down, he'll start eating grass. **He's pretty dumb.**

Radio bemba: Radio lips. **Gossip**

Pata de puerco: Pig leg. **Idiot**

Bemba de perro: Dog lips. **Idiot**

Ñame con corbata: Potato with a tie on. **Idiot with a tie on**

On Your Appearance

Esa no tuvo quinces: She never had a sweet fifteen party. **She's fiercely unattractive.**

Tiene el bonito subido: She's got the pretty up. **She's looking good.**

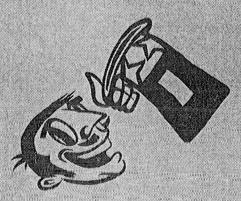

YOU WEAR IT . . . WELL?

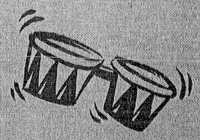

If you've ever met us before, it's safe to say that you've made the assumption that Goodwill and Salvation Army satisfy a good portion of our fashion needs. And you'd be right. Every time we're in one of the thrifts, we invariably start trying to picture the people who once owned the clothes we're sifting through. Most of the time we conjure up images of wildly unusual characters who would have been right at home as extras on the set of *Starsky and Hutch*, but that is just our Huggy-Bear complex. The truth is most of our shirts probably belonged to your dad. You've seen pictures of him in the '70s when he was still macking hard and looking like a cross between the Latin Kojak and the Havana Superfly.

(Thank him for us—those things still need no ironing.)

The reason we bring all this up, of course, is because the subject of this section is clothes, clothes, and more clothes. Just to show you how cemented some of these *ropa* terms are, we challenge you to come up with the proper Spanish for the Spanglish words listed here in less than ten minutes. (Easy you say? You'll see.)

Also, for those of you out there who share our love of thrift shops, we've included our grandmothers' recommendations on whether or not you should buy certain types of used clothing. Enjoy.

suéter n. **a sweater or cardigan**
 Class: Transliteration.
 Origin: Direct phonetic adoption of the English word "sweater."
 Typical usage: "Mira, a ver si te pones el suéter, que el mono está chiflando."

English: "Hey, you better put your *suéter* on because the monkey is whistling. (It's really cold.)

Abuela's Thrifty Tips: Si no tiene mal olor, vale la pena. (If it doesn't stink, it's worth it.)

yin *n.* a pair of jeans
Calbin Clain *n.* Calvin Klein
Doña Karran *n.* Donna Karan

Class: Transliteration.

Origin: Only language came between me and my Calvins.

Typical usage: "*Ni te voy a comprar los yin de Calbin Clain ni de la tal Doña Karran tampoco. Tienes un par de Tofesquin que están nuevo de paquete.*"

English: "I'm not buying you those *yin* from *Calbin Clain,* and I'm not buying the ones from *Doña Karran* either. You've got a pair of Toughskins that are practically new."

blúmer n. women's underwear; panties

Class: Transliteration.

Origin: Taken from the English term "bloomers," which is most often used to refer to young girls' underwear. In a typical Hispanic household, though, full grown women still talk about *"los blúmer que se me perdieron en la secadora."*

Typical usage: "*Muchacha, qué pena he pasado con la visita cuando me di cuenta que la niña dejó unos blúmer sucios en el piso de la sala.*"

English: "My God, I was so embarrassed with my guests when I noticed my daughter left a dirty pair of *blúmer* on the living room floor."

Abuela's *Thrifty Tips: ¿Estarás loca de remate o serás comemierda?* (Are you crazy, or are you just an idiot?)

pántijo n. panty hose

Class: Transliteration.

Origin: A necessary transliteration for ladies shopping at the local drug store.

Typical usage: *¡Saca ese perro, que me va a romper los pántijo!*

English: Get that dog out of here before it rips my panty hose!

pulóver *n.* a T-shirt

Class: Transliteration.

Origin: Adopted from the English term "pullover."

Typical usage: *"Quítate ese pulóver mojado antes que te dé una pulmonía."*

English: "Take off that wet *pulóver* before you catch pneumonia."

tenis *n.* athletic shoes; sneakers

Class: Transliteration.

Origin: Lifted from the first half of "tennis shoes." In English, the word "tennis" is used as an adjective that describes the type of shoes being referred to. However, in Spanish, *"tenis"* takes on the guise of a plural noun and is always paired with an article such as *"los"* or *"unos."* For example, *"pónte unos tenis."*

Typical usage: *"¡Acaba de botar los tenis asquerosos esos que el closet tuyo huele a mierda de elefante, chico!"*

English: "Get rid of those disgusting *tenis* once and for all, man, your closet smells like elephant turds!"

Abuela's Thrifty Tips: *No jodas, si acabo de mandar los tuyos al Gudwil.* (Are you kidding? I just sent yours to Goodwill.)

pansú n. a pantsuit

Class: Transliteration.

Origin: Zayre's clearance rack (non-Miami types: substitute the low-rent store of your choice). Yeah, you remember.

Typical usage: *"Cuando yo llegué a este país y no tenía dinero, me ponía ese pansú tanto que salía caminando solo."*

English: "When I got to this country and had

no money, I used to wear that *pansú* so much that it used to walk on its own."

chor *n.* a pair of shorts

Class: Transliteration.

Origin: Take a wild guess.

Typical usage: "*Óigame, señorita, usted no sale de esta casa con esos chor puestos.*"

English: "Excuse me, little lady, but you're not leaving this house wearing those *chor*."

Abuela's *Thrifty Tips: Se parecen a los que se ponía tu abuelo durante la época de Ford.* (They look like the ones your Grandpa used to wear during the Ford era.)

esmoquin *n.* a tuxedo

Class: Transliteration.

Origin: A phonetic adoption taken from the English term "smoking jacket." Presumably, the connection is in the similarities between a tux jacket and what is commonly referred to as a smoking jacket. Nonetheless, this is an incorrectly adopted term that became accepted through repeated usage.

Typical usage: "*Si la fiesta es de esmoquin yo no voy, vieja.*"

English: "If the party is an *esmoquin* affair, I'm not going, Ma."

Abuela's Thrifty Tips: Si te sirve, cómpralo, porque sale más barato que alquilarlo. (If it fits, buy it. It's cheaper than a rental.)

yaqui *n.* a jacket or windbreaker

Class: Transliteration.

Origin: Taken from "jacket" (as if you couldn't figure it out). It's interesting to note that *yaqui* usually refers to a jacket that protects you from the cold, not one that is part of a suit (*traje*) or a sportcoat (*bléiser*).

Typical usage: "*Primera y última vez que llevo este yaqui a la tintorería; me ha costado un ojo de la cara.*"

English: "That's the first and last time I take this *yaqui* to the cleaners—it cost me an eye off my face."

Abuela's *Thrifty Tips: Tiene un hueco en la manga.* (It's got a hole in the sleeve.)

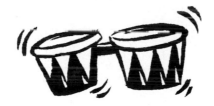

Lost in Translation No. 2

Have you ever paused midsentence to realize that some of the things that come out of your mouth make very little sense to anyone not raised in your cultural pocket? Observe:

Me cayó de lo más bien.	He fell on me well.
¡Vaya, qué clase de aguacero!	Go, what a class of waterzero!
Mira cómo le saca fiesta.	Look at how she's taking a party out of him.
Me están corriendo tremenda máquina.	They're running tremendous machine on me.
Ya me tiene el moño virado.	Now she has my bun twisted.
¡Eso sí que le zumba el mango!	That really lobs the mango!
¡Imagínate tú!	Imagine yourself!
Dímelo cantando.	Tell it to me singing.
Óyeme, ponte para tu número.	Listen, put yourself to your number.
De verdad que estás en lo último.	Truthfully, you are in the last.

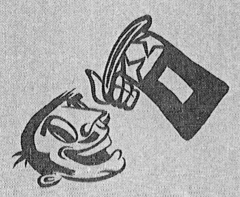

VAIQUAICHON

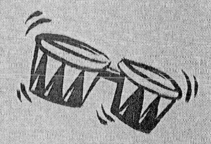

Okay. It's summer. Time to stuff your whole family into the world's smallest hotel room on Miami Beach. Bring Tía Lola, the Hitachi, and the dominos.

Cayo Hueso n. Key West

    Class: Modified transliteration.

    Origin: Cayo is the Spanish word for "key" and "cay," two English words that basically mean the same thing: a small, low island. The twist comes with the word "hueso," which means "bone" in English, but is similar to "west" in its pronunciation. Thus, *Cayo Hueso* could be someone's attempt at a correct translation, but ends up half wrong because of the phonetically based method used to derive the equivalent of "west" in Spanish. The other argument is that since the Spaniards originally colonized the region, it is English speakers who are actually guilty of the erroneous translation. We'll leave it up to you.

Typical usage: "*Cuando me gane el Lotto, voy a vender la casa de perro ésta y nos vamos a Cayo Hueso pa' vivir como marimberos.*"

English: "When I win the lottery, I'm going to sell this doghouse and we're going to *Cayo Hueso* to live like mack daddies."

Guáchinton n. Washington, D.C.

Class: Transliteration.

Origin: Millions of citizenship tests and a mother tongue that makes the pronounciation of the W sound like a G.

Typical usage: The capital of the United States is Guáchinton, D.C.

el súper n. superintendent

Class: Modified transliteration.

Origin: 1970s New York apartment buildings.

Typical usage: Call *el súper* because the garbage disposal just exploded again.

rentar v. to rent property

Class: Modified transliteration.

Origin: Taken from the English word "rent" and modified into Spanish verb form.

Typical usage: "¿Cuánto costará rentar un Yesquí de esos?"

English: "I wonder how much it costs to *rentar* one of those Jet Skis?"

Mallamibish n. Miami Beach

Class: Transliteration.

Origin: We won't insult your intelligence.

Typical usage: "¿Es verdad que compró una casa en Mallamibish el tipo que hizo el papel de Rambo?"

English: "Is it true that the guy who did *Rambo* bought a house in *Mallamibish?*"

> ## *Not To Be Confused*
>
> *guauguau* (dog, usually a puppy) vs. *guagua* (bus)
> *estar arrancando* (kicking ass) vs. *estar arrancado* (broke)

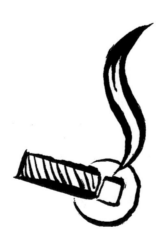

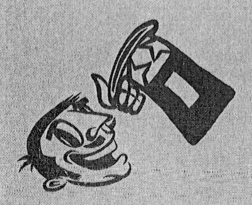

9 TO 5

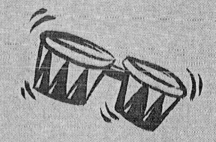

Here's proof that business can be done in more than one language, as you enter the world of *mitins, Guindos,* and *el manayer.*

printear v. **to print; use of a computer printer**
>   *Class:* Modified transliteration.
>   *Origin:* Taken from the English word "print" and converted into "Spanish" form.
>   *Typical usage:* "*Desenchufla la batidora, necesito printear un documento.*"
>   *English:* "Unplug the blender from the wall socket, I've got to *printear* a document."

faxear v. **to fax**
>   *Class:* Modified transliteration.
>   *Origin:* A word adopted from English when there was no common Spanish term for the fax machine.

Typical usage: "*Oye, cuelga el teléfono que te voy a faxear la lista de los vinos cubanos.*"

English: "Hey, hang up the phone, I'm going to *faxear* you the list of Cuban wines."

íncontas adj. Income Tax

Class: Transliteration.

Origin: Come April 15, Latinos across the nation line up and begrudgingly do their duty, leading to this one word modification.

Typical usage: Tell Bebo that I'm going to *filear* him *como un* dependent *en mi íncontas.*

Guindos '95 n. Operating system used on most personal computer systems

Class: Transliteration.

Origin: Redmond, Washington.

Typical usage: "*¿Ese bebito que baila funciona en Guindos '95?*"

English: "Does that dancing baby run on *Guindos '95?*"

Maquintoch n. Operating system used if you're not running *Guindos '95*

    Class: Transliteration.

    Origin: Steve Jobs' housekeeper.

    Typical usage: "*¿Dónde se encuentra el beibi bailarín en tu Maquintoch?*"

    English: "Where can I find the dancing baby on your *Maquintoch?*"

mítin n. a business meeting

    Class: Transliteration.

    Origin: As Latinos joined the American workplace, *una cita* (a meeting) just didn't really feel right, with its images of a real formal affair. Thus was born *el mítin,* a roll-up-your-sleeves-and-get-to-work version of *la cita.*

    Typical usage: Hurry up with the report *que tengo un mítin a las tres.*

bisne n. a business or business endeavor

    Class: Transliteration.

    Origin: The English word "business."

Typical usage: "*Olvídate de la antropología. En esta casa no vas a estar entrando huesos de dinosaurio. Así que cambia el* major *tuyo a* bisne, *que te puede servir para algo.*"

English: "Forget about studying anthropology. You're not bringing any dinosaur bones in this house. You better change your major to something useful like *bisne*."

partain *n.* a part-time job

Class: Transliteration.

Origin: Straight transliteration of the English phrase "part-time." (By the way, if you're lucky, a *partain* leads to a *fultain*.)

Typical usage: "*Mira a ver si te buscas un partain este verano que te veo muy sonso y vago, para no decirte comemierda.*"

English: "See if you can't find yourself a *partain* this summer, because you look a little befuddled and lazy to me. Or should I just call you an idiot?"

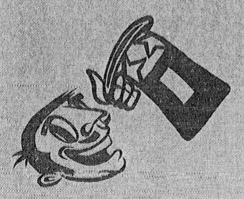

SPORTS

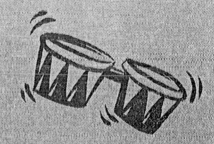

Hispanics love to adapt words from English and make them their own and you'll see that the following terms are no exception. (And after all, "swoosh" is really an international language.) Miami postscript: Jack Ramsay, the Miami Heat's color man, has also made an interesting contribution to linguistics with his addition of the "er" to most basketball shots and moves, producing such great commentary as, "And there's Alonzo Mourning with the left-handed hooker!" Hmm . . . you don't see a lot of those, Dr. Jack.

béisbol n. baseball
jonrón n. a homerun
estraique n. a strike

piche n. a baseball pitcher

Class: Transliteration.

Origin: All phonetic adoptions taken from English terms used in the game of baseball.

Typical usage: "*El juego de béisbol de ayer fue una porquería. El piche de nosotros tenía más chance de sonar un jonrón que de tirar un estraique.*"

English: "Yesterday's *béisbol* game was garbage. Our *piche* had a better chance of hitting a *jonrón* than throwing an *estraique*."

fútbol n. football
fombo n. a fumble
tochdaun n. a touchdown
kique n. placekicker

Class: Transliteration.

Origin: Phonetic adoptions taken from English terms used in the game of football.

Typical usage: "*Ese kique no sirve, chico. Cada vez que toca el fútbol, suelta un fombo y nos suenan otro tochdaun.*"

English: "That *kique* sucks, man. Every time he touches the *fútbol,* he lets go of a *fombo* and they stick us with another *tochdaun.*"

basque *n.* (1) the game of basketball (2) a basket made in a basketball game
***fau n.* a foul**

Class: Transliteration.

Origin: Phonetic adoptions taken from English terms used in the game of basketball.

Typical usage: "*Yo no sirvo pa'l basque porque me encanta repartir Jau.*"

English: "I wasn't made for *basque.* I like to *fau* too much."

joqui *n.* a jockey

Class: Transliteration.

Origin: Taken straight from the American horse's mouth.

Typical usage: "*Ese caballo fue una estafa. Es más que el joqui enano ese no vale quilo.*"

English: "That horse was a gyp. What's more, that midget *joqui* ain't worth a penny."

gol *n.* goal

Class: Transliteration.

Origin: Thanks to transplanted Europeans in America, *fútbol,* or soccer, took hold as a national pastime, resulting in Andrés Cantor's claim to fame.

Typical usage: ¡GGGGGOOOOOOOOOOO OLLLLLLLL! ¡Tremendo golazo! ¡Golazo sensacional!

English: GGGGGOOOOOOOOOOOOOAL-LLLLLLL!

Lost in Translation No. 3

Try to match your favorite American cartoon character to their Hispanic alter ego

1) Trucutú   a. Jughead

2) Casparín (el fan-   b. The Smurfs
   tasma amistoso)

3) Tito   c. Alley Oop

4) Periquita   d. The Lone Ranger

5) Rico Macpato   e. Casper the
                                        Friendly Ghost

6) Motita   f. Woody Wood-

7) Los Pitufos   pecker

8) Torombolo   g. Sluggo

9) El Llanero   h. Nancy
   Solitario   i. Scrooge McDuck

10) El Pájaro Loco   j. Droopy

ANSWERS: 1) c; 2) e; 3) g; 4) h; 5) i; 6) j;
7) b; 8) a; 9) d; 10) f

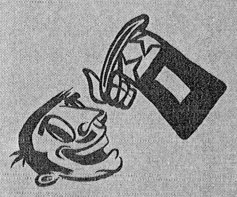

HOME LIFE

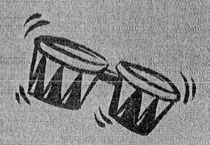

Calabaza, calabaza, *cada uno pa' su casa.* (Pumpkin, pumpkin; everybody go home.) (Don't ask.) Here are some of the things you'll find as you trek through the Spanglish household.

cagüeitin **n. call waiting**
> *Class:* Transliteration.
> *Origin:* That busy signal was multilingual.
> *Typical usage:* "*Te estoy llamando hace media hora pero tu madre no contesta el cagüeitin.*"
> *English:* "I've been calling for half an hour but your mother doesn't answer the *cagüeitin*."

la casita **n. backyard tool shed**
> *Class:* Descriptive.
> *Origin:* Don't think for one second that our

elders didn't know this type of structure was called a "shed." They just got tired of "los americanos" laughing at them because it sounded like they were saying "shit." Their plan: Let's call it *la casita* (little house) and let the gringos figure out what it means.

Typical usage: "*Óyeme lo que te voy a decir, mejor que te pongas para tu número y empieces a fumigar la casita porque acabo de ver una cucaracha del tamaño de un Toyota paseándose por el patio.*"

English: "Listen to me—you'd better get on the ball and get an exterminator for *la casita* because I just saw a cockroach the size of a Toyota parading around our backyard."

londri *n.* laundry

Class: Transliteration.

Origin: Who knew there were so many washer/dryers in the world, much less in America? But with this clear transliteration, Spanish comes clean.

Typical usage: "*No le eche mucho cloro al londri, que la ropa sale dura como un palo.*"

English: "Don't put too much starch in the laundry. It'll turn out hard as a stick."

la secretaria *n.* answering machine

Class: Descriptive.

Origin: In the early '70s, with relatives encountering answering machine messages for largely the first time, this must have seemed funnier than *la maquinita* (the little machine).

Typical usage: "Hello, Lalo, pick up the phone. *Lalo, es tu madre. Bueno,* I can see you have *la secretaria* on."

duple *n.* a duplex

Class: Transliteration.

Origin: Affordable housing, challenging pronunciation.

Typical usage: "*Tengo a mima al lado en el duple y voy a tener que mover la secadora para poner otra puerta.*"

English: "I've got grandma next to my duplex so I'm going to have to move the dryer and install another door."

utíliti *n.* **a utility room**
Class: Modified transliteration.
Origin: As additions were made to the house, this word was added to Latinos' vocabulary.
Typical usage: Búscame el lacasina en el utíliti.
English: Go get me the laquer thinner from the *utíliti*.

lobsí *n.* **the love seat**
Class: Transliteration.
Origin: Keeping up with the Joneses required a household merging of the sofa and the *butaca*.
Typical usage: "Keep an eye on Carmencita, I don't want her and her *quince* partner sitting alone in de *lobsí*."

menteolaten *n.* **Mentholatum**
Class: Transliteration.

Origin: One of the benefits of life in the U.S. is *abuelo* always having this handy.

Typical usage: "Why does *abuela* always smell like *menteolaten.*"

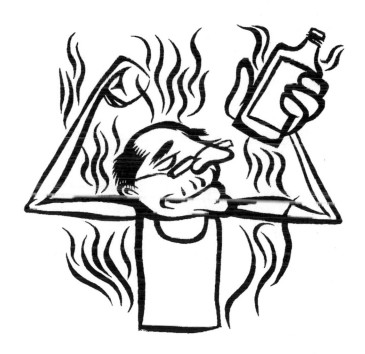

fli *n.* **Raid Ant & Roach Killer**

Class: Descriptive.

Origin: Rather than learning a particular brand name, most Latins opted for this modification of the word "flea," using it as a catch all description for all bug spray.

Typical usage: *"Las hormigas me están matando, hay que comprar fli."*

English: "The bugs are killing me, we've got to buy some *fli.*"

escochteipe *n.* **Scotch Tape**

Class: Transliteration.

Origin: Keeping things together became simplified as Scotch Tape's modified transliteration became a descriptive term used to describe all adhesive tape.

Typical usage: "Bring *abuela* the *escochteipe.* She's mailing a check."

liquiando *v.* **a leak**

Class: Modified transliteration.

Origin: Perhaps because leak described things better than *gotero,* this dramatic word crept into daily usage.

Typical usage: *"¡Apúrate, Pepe, que el techo está liquiando y tengo la casa llena de cubos!"*

English: "Hurry up, Pepe, the roof is *liqui-ando* and my house is full of buckets!"

pipirún *n.* restroom

Class: Descriptive.

Origin: As Latinos having trouble with the word restroom opted for the cuter "pee-pee room," it morphed into this strange but descriptive term, since "pipi" also fills in for certain unmentionable male sex organs.

Typical usage: "Sarita has been in the *pipirún* for hours."

cachumbambé *n.* a see-saw

Class: Traditional.

Origin: Apart from the obviously African construction, unknown.

Typical usage: "*Cachumbambé / la vieja Inés/ que fuma tabaco y toma café.*"

English: "*Cachumbambé / old lady Inés / who smokes cigars and drinks coffee.*" (Cuban folk song.)

Bibaporrú *n.* Vick's VapoRub ointment

Class: Transliteration.

Origin: An oral contraction of the product's name.

Typical usage: Rubbed all over a piece of a paper bag and plastered under your *pulóver* (T-shirt).

jándiman *n.* a handyman

Class: Transliteration.

Origin: Latinos listened to '70s AM radio too.

Typical usage: "*Comma comma comma comma con con / jea, jea, jea / jei beibi / ain jur jándiman.*"

English: See above.

pin pan pun *n.* portable bedding which can be folded for storage purposes; a cot

Class: Descriptive.

Origin: A synopsis of the three-step process associated with the assembly and use of said device. Each syllable is an aural representation of one of the steps, as such: *pin*—the fastener that keeps the bed folded is undone; *pan*—the bed is opened and flattened out; *pun*—you lie down.

Typical usage: "*No seas boba, chica, quédense aquí. Los niños caben en la sofacama y Bebo puede dormir en el pin pan pun.*"

English: "Don't be foolish, girl, you can all stay here. The kids fit on the sofabed and Bebo can sleep on the *pin pan pun*."

floridarrún *n.* **family room of a Hispanic household**

Class: Transliteration.

Origin: Taken from the English term "Florida room."

Typical usage: "*La verdad que las porquerías de la sagüecera no se comparan con los flori-darrún de Hialeah.*"

English: "The truth is those crappy *sagüecera* holes can't compare with any Hialeah *flori-darrún*."

efíchiensi *n.* efficiency housing

Class: Transliteration.

Origin: Even more affordable, still challenging.

Typical usage: "*Mire, señor, estoy buscando una casa con efíchiensi pa' tener un adichional incon.*"

English: "Look sir, I'm looking for a home with an *efíchiensi* so I can have an additional income source."

Fa *n.* Fab laundry detergent

Class: Transliteration.

Origin: Spanish speakers are always tempted by short words that replace longer native equivalents.

Typical usage: "*Bota los pantalones de ese culicagado que ni una caja entera de Fa los limpia.*"

English: "Throw that punk's pants away. Not even an entire box of *Fa* can get them clean."

***pau pau** n.* a spanking

Class: Descriptive / modified transliteration.

Origin: Stems from the English word "pow."
Probably indicative of Hispanics watching a
lot of the old *Batman* TV episodes.

Typical usage: "*Para de decirle que le vas a dar
pau pau. Dile que yo le voy a disparar un so-
plamoco que lo va a dejar pusmao.*"

English: "Stop telling him you're going to
give him *pau pau*. Tell him I'm going to
smack him with a booger-blower that's going
to leave him silly."

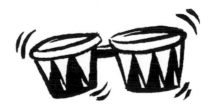

Dad's Favorite Movie Stars

Klin Iswoo	Clint Eastwood
Charle Bronzo	Charles Bronson
Bur Lancaster	Burt Lancaster
Yon Wayne	John Wayne
Bru Li	Bruce Lee
Adi Murfi	Audie Murphy
Chu Norri	Chuck Norris
Yoni Wiesmuler	Johnny Weissmuller
Jonfri Bogar	Humphrey Bogart
Yack Nicelson	Jack Nicholson
(en *Chinataun*)	(in *Chinatown*)

Mom's Favorite Movie Star

Elbi Presli	Elvis Presley

Top 15 household items (circa 1970)

plastic covered furniture*

plastic runner on carpet (the yellow brick road
  of plastic)*

velvet curtains with fringe

El Buddha

ceramic tiger/panther/cat

Santa Bárbara (with occasional offerings)

matador painting

calendar from *el market* (*o farmacia*)

wood panelling

Formica

periquito in a cage

Lladró

plastic fruit

carro de ocho cilindros en el draiwei

espejos everywhere

*Preservation is key.

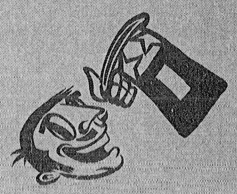

SCIENCE AND
TECHNOLOGY

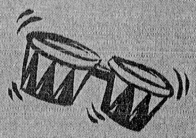

Do you remember the "One of These Things Doesn't Belong" segments from *Sesame Street?* Of course you do. Well, try and take yourself back to the days of Underoos and Silly Putty, and picture the following scenario unfolding on the living room television set: Your *abuelo*. A set of dominoes. A cigar. *Un cafecito.* A lotto ticket. And a VCR. Quick! Which one of these things doesn't belong? Right. Even Big Bird would have said, "*¿Qué carajo pinta Pipo con un VCR, caballeros?*"

It's a glaring truth that Cubans and electronics don't get along very well. This section presents the verbal evidence we have that supports this fact. This is by no means a complete list, but merely a sampling of some of the more colorful highlights. This section would not have been possible without the help of my grandparents—to whom it is dedicated. *Abuela,* I know you meant "synthesizer" when you said *"pianito."* And *Abuelo,* I secretly heeded your warning when you said, *"¡Te vas a volver loco con el Atari ese!"* Well, you were right. *Tenías toda la razón, mi socio.*

celiula *n.* a cellular phone
> *Class:* Transliteration.
> *Origin:* Wireless communication is bilingual.
> *Typical usage: "Voy a tirar la lancha en el canal. Me llevo el celiula por si me empato con un cocodrilo."*
> *English:* "I'm throwing the boat in the canal. I'm taking the *celiula* with me in case I run into a crocodile."

teipear *n.* the act of recording onto an audio cassette or videotape
> *Class:* Modified transliteration.
> *Origin:* The English word "tape" is used as a

root and modified into verb form. Other conjugations include: *teipeando, teipeaste, teipearon, teipéame,* and so on.

Typical usage: "*¡No lo puedo creer, muchacho! ¡Me has borrado la boda de Cuca y Juanito para teipear los salados muñecos amarillos esos!*"

English: "I can't believe it! You erased my tape of Cuca and Juanita's wedding to *teipear* the damned Simpsons!"

tareco *n.* (1) **unidentified electronic device.** (2) **name given to an electronic device during a fit of anger**

Class: Traditional.

Origin: Unknown.

Typical usage: (1) "*Chico, ese bobo de mecánico no tiene ni un pelo. Lo único que sabe hacer es conectar la batería del carro al tareco grande ese, te dice que no sirve y te clava ochenta cocos.*" (2) "*¡Apaga ese tareco de mierda, coño, que me tienes loca!*"

English: (1) "That guy doesn't even have one

mechanic's hair on his head. The only thing he does is hook up the car battery to that big *tareco,* he tells you that it's no good, and then he nails you for eighty bucks." (2) "Turn off that piece of shit *tareco,* damn it, you're driving me crazy!"

bacunclíner *n.* **a vacuum cleaner**

Class: Transliteration.

Origin: It is almost certain that an attempt was made at transliterating "Hoover," but this popular manufacturer's name proved to be quite a challenge. (In Spanish, the "H" would be silent, leaving an awkward double-vowel as the opening syllable sound.) By the time an approximate pronunciation was picked up by ear, it was too late to call it a *júver;* the bag-replacement count on your grandmother's *bacunclíner* was already well into double digits.

Typical usage: "¿Qué fue eso? ¡Ay, coño, el bacunclíner se tragó una pluma!"

English: "What was that? Oh shit, the *bacuncliner* swallowed a pen!"

bíper *n.* a beeper or pager
Class: Transliteration.
Origin: Same place you got your cellular.
Typical usage: "José Ramírez, Chapistería y Jardinero, Teléfono: 555-3196, Bíper: 555-2487."
English: "José Ramírez, Paint and Body Shop and Gardener, Telephone: 555-3196, Bíper: 555-2487.

maicrogüey *n.* a microwave oven
Class: Transliteration.
Origin: Standard phonetic adoption from English.
Typical usage: "Oye, mima, ponme una comida de Weigüiache en el maicrogüey que el bistec empanizado de ayer sabe a palo."
English: "Hey, honey, heat up a Weight Watchers meal for me in the *maicrogüey*— yesterday's breaded steak tastes like a stick."

la jitachi n. **your grandmother's rice cooker**

Class: Transliteration.

Origin: Taken from Hitachi, manufacturer of the omnipotent rice cooker found in many Latino kitchens.

Typical usage: *"Yo no le encuentro la gracia al maicrogüey ese, porque yo puedo usar un tenedor en la jitachi y no explota nada."*

English: "I don't see the point of that microwave, because I can stick a fork in *la jitachi* and nothing explodes."

frijidaire n. **a refrigerator**

Class: Transliteration.

Origin: The Frigidaire Corporation was among the first manufacturers to ship refrigerators to Cuba. Initially, their product was also the most popular of its kind. A Spanish pronunciation was applied to the word that is emblazoned across the product's nameplate, and the proper term *nevera* soon fell by the wayside.

Typical usage: "*Vamos a tener que sacar al lechón del frijidaire, porque la verdad es que tiene una peste que rescucita a Maceo.*"

English: "We're going to have to throw out the roast pig that's in the *frigidaire*. It has a smell that could bring the dead to life."

yombo adj. jumbo sized

Class: Transliteration.

Origin: Dad's attempt to get the most egg for his purchasing dollar.

Typical usage: "I know you want two eggs but with the *yombo* you only need one."

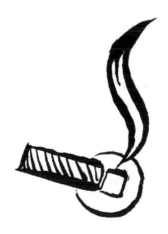

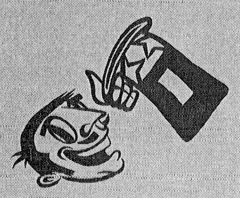

PARDON MOI

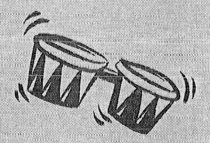

It all began with those darn Chardon designer jeans. "I beg your Chardon" was the ad tag line. When adapting to a foreign culture, you're bound to step on some toes. Here are some words to make it a little less painful.

plis adv. **please**
> *Class:* Transliteration.
> *Origin:* Trying to squeeze your way to the exit door of the subway required this bit of Spanglish.
> *Typical usage: Esquiyesmi. Esquiyesmi, plis.*

esquiyesmi adv. **excuse me**
> *Class:* Modified transliteration.

Origin: That same subway.

Typical usage: See above.

sori *adv.* **Sorry**

Class: Transliteration.

Origin: Stepping on a the toes of your Americana girlfriend while at the Hop.

Typical usage: Ayen sori, my darling.

ayen sori con esquiyesmi *adv.* **I'm sorry, excuse me**

Class: Modified transliteration.

Origin: Stepping on a few toes, trying to get off that same subway train. Because "I beg your pardon" was just too hard to pronounce.

Typical usage: Míster, ayen sori con esquiyesmi, míster.

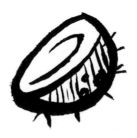

Top 7 names for a dog*

Blackie
King
Champion
Lulú
Chuchi
Rocky
Baby

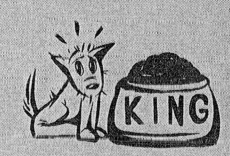

Top name for a cat

Miso (or Misu, depending on your geographic location)

*Remember, these are pronounced with a Spanish accent.

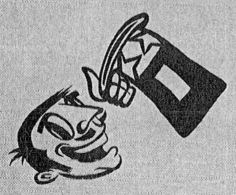

PUT IT IN YOUR MOUTH

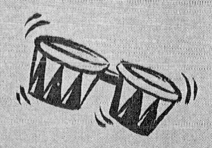

Hispanics give new meaning to the term Food and Drug Administration. Here's some gourmet slang we love to spit out.

lonchando v. having lunch

Class: Modified transliteration.

Origin: In the name of efficiency and speed, Cubans will occasionally concede to Anglos and replace a Spanish word with a variant of a more nimble English equivalent. Here are the numbers: *Almorzando* (proper term)—4 syllables, 0.6 seconds conversation time. *Lonchando*—3 syllables, 0.4 seconds conversation time. We have a winner.

Typical usage: *"Dile que estoy lonchando.*
No tengo ganas de hablar con el antipático ese."
English: "Tell him I'm *lonchando*. I don't feel
like talking to that lame-ass."

cachú *n.* **tomato ketchup**
Class: Transliteration.
Origin: Do you realize what the word Heinz
looked like to native Spanish speakers? Nei-
ther did they.
Typical usage: *"No botes los paqueticos de*
cachú, muchacho. Se ve que tú no sabes lo
que es trabajar por el dinero."
English: "Don't throw away those little pack-
ets of *cachú*, young man! You don't
know what it is to have to work for your
money."

güaquer *n.* **Quaker Oats brand cereal**
Class: Transliteration.
Origin: This product, when compared to cold
cereal, differs significantly in terms of tex-

ture and method of preparation. Therefore, Hispanics do not include it in the cold cereal blanket category of *confley* (see entry below). It is the sole exception to the "everything is *confley*" rule.

Typical usage: "*A la vieja mía se le cayó un plato de qüaquer hoy y ha formado una clase de cagazón en la alfombra que eso no tiene nombre.*"

English: "My old lady dropped a plate of *qüaquer* on the rug today and made a mess of shit that has no name."

confley *n.* any kind of dry breakfast cereal

Class: Transliteration.

Origin: Taken from the English words "corn flakes" and used as a category-wide reference. Remember, it can be Fruity Pebbles, Trix, Cocoa Puffs, or Raisin Bran and it's still *confley.*

Typical usage: "*¡Carajo! Lo primero que hace este muchacho es meter la mano en la* *caja de confley para sacar el juguete de mierda.*"

English: "Damn it! The first thing he does is stick his weaselly little hand into the cereal box so he can get that little toy."

quei *n.* a cake

Class: Transliteration.

Origin: Once again, we have an example of an English word providing the fuel for the rapid-fire verbal style Hispanics have perfected. You can't beat one syllable.

Typical usage: "*Cincuenta bocaditos . . . cincuenta cangrejitos . . . cincuenta croqueticas . . . y un quei para cincuenta personas.*"

English: "Fifty finger sandwiches . . . fifty crab pastries . . . fifty little croquettes . . . and a *quei* for fifty people." (Taken from a popular Spanish-radio ad campaign for a Cuban bakery in Miami. We never really understood it either.)

petipuá *n.* green peas

Class: Transliteration.

Origin: Taken from the French words *"petit pois,"* meaning "small peas."

Typical usage: *"¡Que no le saques los petipuá al arroz con pollo, te he dicho!"*

English: "I said not to take the *petipuas* out of the *arroz con pollo!"*

jambergue *n.* a hamburger

Class: Transliteration.

Origin: Not yet known. We will have an answer when the age-old debate between Cuban exiles and their children is resolved, i.e., which came first: McDonald's or *Fritas Dominó?*

Typical usage: *"Claro, te comiste las papitas, pero has dejado el jambergue muerto de la risa."*

English: "Sure, you ate all your french fries, but you left the *jambergue* laughing at you on your plate."

Jamón del Diablo n. **Underwood deviled-ham product**

Class: Descriptive.

Origin: Reference to the little red devil that appears on the white product label.

Typical usage: "No te pongas a ordenar pastelitos. Tráeme cinco laticas de Jamón del Diablo y dos paquetes de queso crema y yo te preparo unos bocaditos que son una delicia."

English: "Don't go and order pastries. Bring me five cans of *Jamón del Diablo* and two packages of cream cheese and I'll make some kick-ass little sandwiches."

wisqui n. **whiskey**

Class: Transliteration.

Origin: The drink of choice besides rum in Latin society, and a transliteration as old as the hills.

Typical usage: "Listen, son, you can't sit at the bar with me and order those drinks with the umbrellas in them. *Los hombres toman wisqui* [real men drink whiskey]."

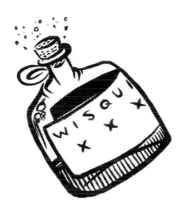

beicon *n.* bacon

Class: Transliteration.

Origin: Straight phonetic adoption.

Typical usage: "*El año pasado el médico me quitó el beicon. Ahora me quitan el wisqui. Lo único que se queda es que me quiten el culo para no poder cagar más.*"

English: "Last year the doctor took the *beicon* away. Now, he says no *wisqui*. All I need now is for him to take my ass away and leave me with no way to take a dump."

péter n. any chocolate candy bar

Class: Transliteration.

Origin: American candymaker Peter Paul was among the first to ship individually wrapped chocolate bars to Cuba. For exiled Cubans, the first half of the brand name went on to become a generic term for all of the products in this category, that is, Nestlé Crunch = *péter,* Three Musketeers = *péter,* Sweet Temptations Fat-Free Chocolate Bar = *péter seco* (dry péter), and so on.

Typical usage: "*Vieja, sabía yo que te iba a entrar tremenda flojera con el péter que te jamastes.*"

English: "Ma, I knew you would end up getting the runs with that *péter* you munched down."

cuqui (1) *adj.* kooky (2) *n.* a cookie (3) *n.* a nickname for a sweet girl

Class: Modified transliteration.

Origin: Proper swinging to the Rat Pack required this transliteration best exemplified in tío Manny's reading of Sinatra's *The Lady Is a Tramp*.

Typical usage: (1) "She loves that free, fresh, crazy, *cuqui* wind in her hair."

(2) "Don't feed the dog any more of my sugar *cuquis!*"

(3) "Go check on *Cuqui* and her date. I think they might be sitting on the *lobsí*."

yogur *n.* yogurt

Class: Transliteration.

Origin: As the health food craze of the '80s took hold, Latinos discovered this European treat. And this was even before Hispanic-friendly flavors like mamey and guava were introduced.

Typical usage: "Ever since *Abuela's* teeth fell out, all she wants to eat is *yogur*."

Hotdo *n.* a frankfurter

Class: Transliteration.

Origin: Adapting to life in America, hot dog became *hotdo* and *apelpai* meant apple pie.

Typical usage: see *Sebenileben,* page 41.

transén *n.* a Tranxene sedative in pill form

Class: Transliteration.

Origin: An off-the-label phonetic adoption of the name of a respected wonder drug that miraculously diminishes, suppresses, and otherwise curtails murderous impulses in middle-aged Cuban women.

Typical usage: "*Oye, mijita, no te alteres. Tómate un transén, que la cosa se va a poner fea.*"

English: "Listen, girl, don't get stressed out. Pop a *transén,* or things are gonna get ugly."

bistec *n.* a steak; usually of the palomilla variety

Class: Transliteration.

Origin: Derived orally from the English term "beefsteak." (It is worth noting that this word

is often erroneously acknowledged as a
"true" Spanish word.)

Typical usage: *"¡Coño, mima, el bistec está más frío que un sapo ruso!"*

English: "Damn, woman! This *bistec* is colder than a Russian toad!"

sángüiche n. a sandwich

Class: Transliteration.

Origin: The Latin American cafés around the United States.

Typical usage: *"Ya te dije que en un minuto sale el sángüiche cubano especial; trágate un transén y no me jodas más, chico."*

English: "I already told you that the special cuban *sángüiche* is coming out in a minute; take a Tranxene and get off my ass, buddy!"

Lost in Translation No. 4

Match these ñ foods to their American
cousins.

1) *merenguitos*   a. tasty Spam

2) *fritas*   b. Dr. Pepper

3) *buñuelos*   c. vanilla pudding
                                 with texture

4) *batido de mamey*   d. mashed yams

5) *churros*   e. strawberry Quik

6) *carne fría*   f. donuts with pan-
                                 cake syrup

7) *coditos*   g. cranberry paste
                                 in a box

8) Iron Ber   h. Cool Whip

9) *galleticas de María*   i. porkburgers

10) *dulce de guayaba*   j. elephant ears

11) *arroz con leche*   k. Hamburger Helper

12) *fufú*   l. graham crackers

ANSWERS: 1) h; 2) i; 3) f; 4) e; 5) j; 6) a;
7) k; 8) b; 9) l; 10) g; 11) c; 12) d

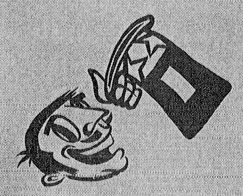

BEER

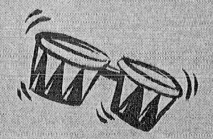

Cerveza is a constant in American culture. Hispanic culture, too. In fact, we can't think of one where it ain't. When you need a frosty one but you can't pronounce the name, the only thing to do is get creative with the label.

Llave n. a Beck's beer

Class: Descriptive.

Origin: The small key (or *llave*) that decorates the label on bottles of Beck's is the source of this reference.

Typical usage: "*¿Cuatro pesos por una Llave? No jodas, chico, tráeme una Budweiser.*"

English: "Four bucks for a *Llave*? Screw that, buddy, get me a Budweiser."

muñequita *n.* a St. Pauli Girl beer consumed by a Hispanic

Class: Descriptive.

Origin: The literal meaning of this Spanish word, "little doll," is a reference to the maiden depicted on the bottle's label.

Typical usage: "*Dáme un paquete de Malboro y una muñequita para mojarme la bemba.*"

English: "Gimme a pack of Marlboro, and a *muñequita* to wet my lips."

Indio Sudado *n.* An Hatuey Beer

Class: Descriptive

Origin: The traditional Cuban beer, now brought back to life in Miami, features Native hero Hatuey on its package. This Cuban Indian told the Spanish where to put their hops, so to speak, and the sweaty part refers to condensation.

Typical usage: Nena, ve te a la nevera en el patio y traeme un Indio Sudado.

English: Nena, go to the freezer and get me an *Indio Sudado.*

Estrellita *n.* Heineken

Class: Descriptive

Origin: Earned its Spanish moniker for the star on its label or cap when it's imported directly from Europe.

Typical Usage: La Estrellita de Europa es mucho mas fuerte que la de aqui.

English: La Estrellita from Europe is much stronger than the one from here.

El Oso Sudado *n.* Cold Polar Beer

Class: Descriptive.

Origin: An ice-cold polar beer has been thus named for the polar-bear logo on the bottle, covered with heavy condensation.

Typical Usage: Tomo el oso para mear sabroso.

English: Drink the bear if you wanna pee with flavor. (Not very funny, but in Spanish it rhymes, kind of like, "If it's clear, it's beer."

El Toro n. Schlitz Malt Liquor

Class: Descriptive

Origin: Latinos slowly discovered the stronger effects of malt liquor, and indeed, no one does it like the bull.

Typical Usage: El toro este sabe a Windex pero te de tremenda nota.

English: This *El Toro* tastes like Windex, but it gets me horned out.

Cabeza de perro n. Guinness

Class: Descriptive.

Origin: Forget pronouncing Guinness, and with that scary dog head on the label, who would call it anything else? Known in the Latin community for the dog head as well as for its rumored aphrodisiac effects.

Typical Usage: La verdad es que la cabeza de perro me tiene a mil.

English: The truth is this dog's head has me going a million miles an hour.

Medical Conditions

cólico: colic, soothed only by *tilo* and mom's incessant hovering.

destemplanza: a little bit of fever, enough to send *abuela* into a tizzy, but not enough to actually register on a thermometer. How is it measured? With *abuela's* curious gaze and a clammy hand to the forehead. Accuracy is irrelevant.

patatún: unexplainable, unavoidable collapse. Similar to *embolia,* but different.

embolia: neuro-muscular shutdown, usually instigated by the much-warned-against swim-after-eating. Also see *patatún.*

tener un peo: sloppy-ass drunk.

sentirse campana: feeling A-okay.

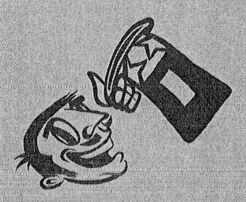

ESTO Y OTRO
(DIS & DAT)

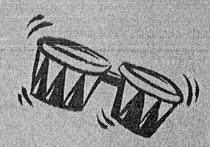

Think back to the last time you heard someone use the phrase "What a pass!" Was it last month? Yesterday? Maybe five minutes ago? (Actually, if it was five minutes ago, there's a good chance you are walking through Miami's Westland Mall right now.) No matter, as a member of generation ñ, you know exactly what it means: *"Oye, te las pasaste."* (You went too far.) There are two characteristics that distinguish "a pass" from other Cuban-Americanisms. First, it takes a word from Spanish and converts it into an Englishlike phrase—that's the reverse of what we've seen so far. Second, and most important, your Tío Manolito didn't come up with it. We came up with it. Maybe not you and us specifically, but a lot of these are most definitely the work of a fellow ñ-er. Other ones come from the fact that Latinos have trouble with the "w" sound. And some are just plain too weird to leave out.

estop 1. *v.* to stop 2. *n.* stop sign
 Class: Transliteration.
 Origin: Caution sign painted on Hispanic ice cream vendor's truck.
 Typical Usage: (1) Children. Estop. Eslow. (2) "Ese cabrón se llevó el estop y por poquito me hace tiza."
 English: (2) "That S.O.B. ran the *estop* and almost made me into chalk! (almost killed me!)"

guau adj. wow
 Class: Transliteration.
 Origin: The first thing said by the first Latino to arrive in Vegas.
 Typical usage: "¡Guau!"
 English: "Wow!"

chou adj. to make a scene

Class: Descriptive.

Origin: Perhaps "He made a scene" was too vague, or just not emphatic enough for Hispanics, who opted to create an entire show instead of just one scene.

Typical usage: "El parti estaba divertidísimo, pero tu conoces a tu tío: armó tremendo chou."

English: "The party was going great, but then—you know your uncle—he staged a big chou."

jiti n. A smack

Class: Descriptive.

Origin: Your eloquent older brother.

Typical usage: "Estás brincando en el trampolín de la confianza y vas a caer en la piscina del jiti."

English: "You're bouncing on the trampoline of informality and you're about to land in the pool of smacks."

roquenrol *adj.* Rock 'n' Roll

    Class: Modified transliteration

    Origin: 1956: Elvis appears on *The Ed Sullivan Show.* Elvis is everywhere.

    Typical usage: "I lof roquenrol."

roquero *adj.* a Rock 'n' Roll dude

    Class: Modified transliteration.

    Origin: Oh, maybe the Mexican band Mana.

    Typical usage: "¡Yo sé que tú eres roquero pero con ese pelo largo tienes una pinta de buscanovio!"

    English: "I know that you're a rocker but with that long hair you look like you're looking for a boyfriend."

japiverdei *n.* a birthday

    Class: Modified transliteration.

    Origin: "Japiverdei tu ju . . . Japiverdei tu ju . . ."

    Typical usage: "Ven por la casa que hoy es el japiverdei de Jerri y le vamos a cortar un quei."

    English: "Come by the house because today

is Jerry's *japiverdei* and we're gonna have some cake."

yanqui n. an Anglo; English-speaker born in the United States

Class: Transliteration.

Origin: Fear of cultural imperialism.

Typical usage: "*Estos yanquis tienen cada cosa.*"

English: "These *yanqui* folk have their weird ways."

caché adj. cachet

Class: Transliteration.

Origin: Oh, French words get transliterated too—these guys will appropriate anything.

Typical usage "*A ella tú la ves con sus años avanzados y no te puedes imaginar el caché ella tenía.*"

English: "You see her with her advanced years, and you can hardly imagine the *caché* she had in her day."

foni *adj.* **funny, not ha-ha funny, just funny**

Class: Transliteration.

Origin: The wildly popular syndicated bilingual TV show, *¿Qué Pasa USA?*

Typical usage: "Don't get sonny with me *foni*-boy!"

English: One and the same.

embarkation *n.* **failure in adhering to a previous commitment or agreement**

Class: Modified transliteration.

Origin: After experiencing some sort of letdown, most of us switch over to Spanish and exclaim, "*¡Coño, tremendo embarque!*" And let's face it, no phrase in English was as effective, direct, and succinct as this one until we came up with . . .

Typical usage: "Shit, bro, tremendous *embarkation!*"

lonplei *n.* **a long playing vinyl record album**

Class: Transliteration.

Origin: Abbey Road

Typical usage: "*Estoy buscando el lonplei de los Bétal donde salen vestido de conejos.*"

English: "I'm looking for the *lonplei* by the Beatles where they appear dressed as bunnies." (*Magical Mystery Tour*)

guei adj. gay

Class: Transliteration.

Origin: Politically correct Latinos opted for this one over *pato.*

Typical usage: "*Qué nice es ese muchacho, pero creo que el es un poco guei.*"

English: "He's a nice boy, but I think he's a little *guei.*"

cag(1.) *n.* improbable outcome attributable to good fortune (2.) *v.* the act of transforming an improbability into a reality by invoking the powers of random chance

Class: Modified transliteration.

Origin: Almost certainly born in the high-school basketball courts of Miami, "cag" is the language-hopping derivative of the Spanish phrase *"te cagaste,"* which translates into "you shit your pants." The meaning implied is this: "You have no idea what just happened. It was out of your hands and you should be embarrassed." For example, a pass intended as a fastbreak that ends up swooshing through the net for three undeserved points is a "cag" of the highest order. In a similar vein, everything that ever happened to Mr. Magoo could be considered a cag.

Typical usage: 1. "Oh my God! What a cag! ¡*Límpiate!*" 2. "Okay, 9-ball in the side pocket . . . no, wait . . . in the . . . forget it, man, I'm just gonna cag it."

enpingated adj. empowered by extreme anger
   Class: Modified transliteration.
   Origin: Sorry, but if you're not familiar with the profane Spanish word this stems from, we're not going to elaborate here. (We're try-

ing to maintain a family-publication feel, you know.)

Typical usage: "Roly me va a tener enpingated if he embarkates again, bro."

English: "Roly is going to get me *enpingated* if he sells out again, bro."

fuácata *adj.* state of being broke

Class: Descriptive.

Origin: Too much time on their hands. This word arose from different ways of describing poverty in Cuba.

Typical usage: "Estoy en la fuácata como una puta en cuaresma" or *"Estoy en la fuácata tan dura que me estoy comiendo un chino crudo"* or *"Estoy en la fuácata que estoy paseando la Niagara en bicicleta."*

English: "I'm in the *fuácata* like a hooker during Lent" or "I'm in the *fuácata* so hard I'm eating a raw Asian person" or "I'm in the *fuácata* so hard I'm navigating Niagara Falls on a bike."

miamijapi adj. **Feeling of joy experienced by World Series Champs the Florida Marlins**

> *Class:* It's just not clear.
>
> *Origin:* State of euphoria descending upon Florida Marlins' pitcher and MVP Liván Hernández.
>
> *Typical usage:* When asked how he felt about winning the World Series, Hernández replied: "Miamijapi, me japi, manager japi, everybody japi!"
>
> *English:* That was English.

bisi adj. **busy; occupied**

> *Class:* Transliteration.
>
> *Origin:* Taken from the English word "busy."
>
> *Typical usage:* "*Tu abuela también está bisi, pero ella sí tiene tiempo para llamarte a tí.*"
>
> *English:* "Your grandmother is *bisi* too, but she has time to call."

flonquear v. **to fail an examination or course**

> *Class:* Modified transliteration.
>
> *Origin:* A phonetic adoption of the En-

glish term "flunk" modified into Spanish verb form.

Typical usage: "*¡Suelta el teléfono ya, que vas a flonquear el año y te lo juro que te quedas aquí con tu abuela cuando nos vayamos a Cayo Hueso la semana que viene!*"

English: "Let go of the telephone already—you're going to *flonquear* the school year and I swear you'll stay home with your grandmother when we go to Key West next week!"

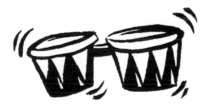

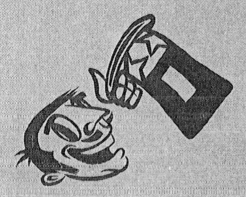

AMERICRISMAS

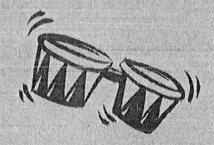

"Big Man, you been rehearsing real hard so Santa will bring you a new saxophone?" was the musical question Bruce Springsteen asked in his inspired version of "Santa Claus Is Coming to Town." The Boss rules, but he's not the only one who rocks at Christmas time. Hispanics like to groove to their own jingle bells, and even Phil Spector's *A Christmas Gift for You* doesn't compare to the Salsoul Orchestra's *Disco Christmas*. Here's what happens when the Spanglish yuletide comes in.

americrismas adj. + n. holiday greeting exchanged among Spanish speakers; *syn. Merry Christmas*

Class: Transliteration.

Origin: José Feliciano.

Typical usage: "*¡Ay guana güich ju ameri-crismas!*"

English: See above.

frizando *v.* **to make frozen; freezing**

Class: Modified transliteration.

Origin: Taken from the English word "freeze" and modified into mock Spanish.

Typical usage: "*Que será de la vida de Alina en New Jersey. Imagínate, se estará frizando las nalgas y cagándose en el día que se fue de Miami.*"

English: "I wonder how things are going for Alina in New Jersey. I guess she must be *frizando* her ass off and cursing the day she left Miami."

Santiclós *n.* **the Cuban Santa Claus**

Class: Transliteration.

Origin: The current incarnation of Kris

Kringle's Hispanic alias is actually a revision of a previous name given to him. Originally, most Latins adopted him as a saint. In those days, he was *San Ticlós*, as many elders will recount. Exactly when he lost his saintlihood is uncertain, but we're sure those Claymation prime-time TV specials had something to do with it.

Typical usage: "*¡Sigue portándote mal! ¡Ojalá que Santiclós te deje un mojón más grande que tu cabeza!*"

English: "Go ahead, keep misbehaving. I hope *Santiclós* brings you a turd bigger than your head!"

San Guíbin *n.* **patron saint of pilgrims born on the last Thursday in November**

Class: Transliteration.

Origin: Derived from "Thanksgiving." The American national holiday was transformed into a person of holy stature by Spanish-speaking Catholics eager for a new saint to petition. Though the fictional *San Guíbin* seems to have secured a celestial post in Hispanic culture, an air of doubt has always lingered due to the curious absence of an *estampita* (prayer stamp). And, admittedly, that rotating birthday thing looks kind of suspicious.

Typical usage: "Ay, niña, ¿quién te mandaría a empatarte con un novio americano? Ahora hay que cocinar dos pavos de San Guíbin: uno con mojo y el otro reseco."

English: "Girl, who told you to go out and get an American boyfriend? Now we have to cook two *San Guíbin* turkeys: one with mojo sauce and the other dry as hell."

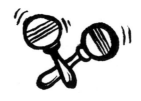

And Just in Time for the Holidays . . .

Merry Matching to You and to All a *Buenas Noches*

The Traditional	Our House
turkey	*lechón*
prayer before eating	drunken tirade against Castro
caroling in your neigh-borhood	screaming across the table
Christmas morning gift giving	countdown to midnight
dinner rolls	*pan cubano*
potatoes	*yuca*
stuffing	rice and beans
fruit cake	*turrón*
Have you been a good boy/girl this year?	*¿Cuántas novias/novios tú tienes?*

Most Lovable Christmas Character

Traditional	ñ
Rudolph the Red Nosed Reindeer	El Burrito Sabanero
Kris Kringle (Jolly gift-giving old man)	Tío Manolo, *el marimbero* (jolly gift-giving old man)
Frosty the Snow Man (melts in the sunshine)	*el primo* from New Jersey (burns in the sunshine)
Ebenezer Scrooge, Bah Humbug man	Lalo, *el vecino aguafiestas*